In her career as a journalist, Susan Wyndham has been editor of *Good Weekend* magazine, New York correspondent for *The Australian* newspaper, and literary editor and deputy editor of *The Sydney Morning Herald*. She is currently a senior writer for the *Herald* and lives in Sydney with her husband.

Life In His Hands

The True Story of a
Neurosurgeon and a Pianist

SUSAN WYNDHAM

For Liz,

The story of two more
people who never give
up. Very best wishes

Susan Wyndham

PICADOR
Pan Macmillan Australia

First published 2008 in Picador by Pan Macmillan Australia Pty Limited
1 Market Street, Sydney

National Library of Australia
Cataloguing-in-Publication data:

Wyndham, Susan.
Life in his hands/author, Susan Wyndham.
Sydney: Pan Macmillan, 2008.

ISBN: 9781405038379 (pbk.)

Teo, Charles.
Neurosurgeons – Australia – Biography.

617.48092

Every endeavour has been made to contact copyright holders to obtain the necessary
permission for use of copyright material in this book. Any person who may have
been inadvertently overlooked should contact the publisher.

Typeset in 12.5/16 pt Granjon by Midland Typesetters, Australia
Printed in Australia by McPherson's Printing Group

Papers used by Pan Macmillan Australia Pty Ltd are natural, recyclable products made
from wood grown in sustainable forests. The manufacturing processes conform to the
environmental regulations of the country of origin.

CONTENTS

PROLOGUE

Charlie Teo could not find his lucky socks, and without them he couldn't operate. In the chill of the morning he had already paddled his kayak on Sydney Harbour. Nothing calmed his mind and steadied his muscles like the rhythm of slicing into cold, hard water. He had eaten a bowl of muesli; any more food and the blood would rush from his head to his stomach. He prepared for surgery as if he were a sportsman: get the endorphins running, be alert and stay strong.

Charlie Teo had buckets of confidence. He had strong, honey-skinned fingers that could hover over an open brain for hours, cutting and burning without a hint of tremor. His lean figure could be mistaken for flimsy but his calves and forearms bulged and his slight stoop came from the tension of taut muscles. He could stand in the operating theatre for five, ten, twenty hours at a stretch, one foot in its leather clog resting on the other, the only cost a few collapsed veins on his legs.

The house hummed with chatter as Charlie's wife herded their four small daughters into the day. He went upstairs to hunt through his sock drawer. Then he would sit down, tune out the voices from below and breathe deeply. Just a few minutes' solitude: his way of meditating before revving up his motorbike and heading for the operating theatre.

But first he had to find his socks.

Thursday 16 August 2001 was a day he would rather turn his back on. He only had one patient booked for surgery, a young concert pianist, but it would be a long operation, possibly his most difficult. Whatever he might achieve in the coming hours, he didn't expect the pianist ever to play another pure note.

I still have the two pages of scrawl from my first telephone conversation with Charlie Teo. I left him a message in June 2002 saying I wanted to talk about his patient Aaron McMillan for a story in *The Sydney Morning Herald*. When he returned my call at home early one Sunday morning, he wasn't the remote professional I had been expecting. Although I knew nothing about him, doctors, in my experience, were often formal in interviews and suspicious of the media.

'I'm forty-five,' said Charlie. 'I love looking at girls. I have a motorbike. I have no artistic interests. I'm a bit of a philistine and I call a spade a bloody shovel.'

He spoke with passion and put no restrictions on the notes I scribbled sitting on my bed that morning. I liked him immediately, even though I didn't understand why he would offer such a bad-boy sketch of himself to a stranger who was also a journalist. He was equally frank about his work and about

Aaron, the pianist he had operated on ten months earlier for a rare kind of brain tumour.

'He's hard to describe because he's almost unique,' Charlie said. 'When I first met him I thought he was mainly bullshit. No one this age was so mature, so at peace with his position in life and so spiritually grounded. As I get to know him I realise it's not bullshit. He wants to heal the world through music.'

Charlie's bemused admiration fed my own curiosity. In March that year I had been invited to a dinner at New South Wales Parliament House held by the Australian supporters of a new library being built in Egypt on the site of the ancient Library of Alexandria. I spoke for a long time to an Egyptian guest and others at our end of the table. There were speeches. Quite late in the evening I turned to the palely handsome young man on my left.

Aaron had a placid smile and an open manner. He had just turned twenty-five and yet he had an older man's poise. He would admit years later that he had been annoyed at being seated among non-dignitaries, but we made pleasant small talk. Then at last he broke through our politeness to tell me, briefly, about his recent experiences. I had missed the episode of the ABC television program *Australian Story* that had made his drama familiar to almost a million viewers. But he told the story so well that I felt I had left my chair and taken a journey to the blurry edge of life, where he had been. The massive tumour, the risky surgery, the remarkable recovery had brought him here – fresh, healthy and planning to release an album of piano solos later in the year. We agreed to meet again for an interview for *The Sydney Morning Herald*. Perhaps, I thought, he was just a clever self-promoter.

Three months later, Aaron called to say his CD was soon to

be launched and we met in a cafe in my office building. By the time I had sat with him for two hours with a tape recorder, I was intrigued. Despite his youth he could articulate the great questions of life, art and human aspiration. He could talk about the inner workings of his brain. He exuded, at the same time, serenity and impatience to live at double speed. And he *was* a brilliant self-promoter.

The idea for a book took hold as I wrote about Aaron and Charlie in several newspaper articles, and grew to know them as men. They had many similarities. Both mavericks in their fields, they were pungent, inspiring, eloquent, funny and stubborn characters who had confronted death – one of them his own and the other on most days in the operating theatre. They also represented a meeting of opposites: art and science, ethereal and physical, blond and dark good looks. Our conversations carried me into exciting zones of endurance and courage, music and medicine, body and mind, life and death. They gave me an insight into the human brain, the most challenging organ for surgeons, scientists and philosophers.

During my research, I watched Charlie operate and gazed into many brains, learning about their structure, functions and mal-functions. At first I felt dismay that the complex centre of the self was just a bowl of bloody, gelatinous goo, amazement that this pulpy mess could be such a refined instrument of thought and emotion – and relief that I was not going to faint. For all its secret intricacy, a naked brain is somehow less disturbing, less personal, than other viscera. I could watch with detached awe the neuro-surgeon's fancywork. Soon I was hooked on the thrill of brain surgery as others are exhilarated by climbing mountains or paragliding.

The greatest lessons about the mind, however, did not come

from watching a physical organ. When I began the book in early 2003, and even when it was half-written at the end of that year, I thought it was about a medical triumph, aided by extraordinary strength of spirit in both the patient and the doctor. The story formed a neat dramatic arc and ended in success.

As months and then years went by, though, a much more complicated story evolved, about how to live in the face of death. It was not a story I wanted to tell. But by then I was not just on the sidelines; I was racing to keep up with events as they happened around me.

PART ONE

'A musician, if he's a messenger, is like a child who hasn't been handled too many times by man, hasn't had too many fingerprints across his brain.'

Jimi Hendrix

I

BLIND SPOT

Vanity saved Aaron McMillan's life in the winter of 2001. Later there were other, more complex and nobler reasons for his survival; later he could laugh at the trivial portent. But this is how it began.

In those short, dark days, the only thing that mattered to Aaron was finishing his CD of piano music. He was twenty-four and building a reputation as a concert pianist, but he had grander ambitions and this self-produced album was intended to launch him financially.

For now, though, it was costing him a thousand dollars for every late-night session at the Australian Broadcasting Corporation's recording studio, down the dingy end of Sydney near Central Station. He had to work fast. There were twenty-eight tracks, each chosen by a friend or family member. The mood of the music swung from the showy Sonata in C by Scarlatti to Eric Satie's tranquil *Gymnopédie No. 1*, written when the composer was Aaron's age; from the stately Impromptu in A flat, written by Schubert a year before his death at thirty-one, to the haunting Adagio from the *Moonlight Sonata*, in which Aaron sensed the young Beethoven's despair as deafness began to close in on him.

Yossi Gabbay had already done a day's work as a sound engineer for ABC Classic FM on the evenings Aaron arrived, coming out of the cold into the wood-lined cocoon of the Eugene Goossens Hall. They would begin work straight away. Aaron sat alone at the piano, a distinguished 1962 Steinway grand that had been mellowed by masters such as Vladimir Ashkenazy and Roger Woodward, while behind the glass of the control room Yossi turned on the red light and gave a small wave to tell Aaron he was recording. When Aaron thought he hadn't captured a passage or Yossi heard a sound he didn't like, they would speak through the talkback system and begin again. Mostly they pushed on.

As the weeks went by, Yossi noticed that Aaron was stopping more often, sometimes banging the keys in frustration.

'Aaron, it's okay. We can just start again,' he would say.

After twenty-five years in the studio, Yossi knew how to soothe the most temperamental performers. Aaron might lope in wearing jeans, running shoes and an easygoing smile, but underneath he was as driven as any musician Yossi had seen.

Often they worked until midnight, recording then editing. Sometimes Aaron complained that he had a headache and couldn't concentrate, so Yossi would make Turkish coffee and tell him not to get into knots. Most nights they left the studio and walked into Chinatown for a meal, after which Aaron seemed to have energy even for the most difficult pieces he had set himself.

More and more, Aaron just wanted to flop on the black couch

in the studio. If he had tried to describe his suffering, either to Yossi or to himself, he would have said he felt as if someone were slowly turning an egg-beater deep inside his head. Instead, he just knew he had a headache that came and went and was worst when he moved quickly. Tilting to lay his head on the pillow at night was agony and rising from his bed in the morning almost made him collapse. For months he dulled the ache with painkillers and rest. The pain built so gradually that he almost stopped experiencing the familiar sensation as pain.

He'd been having the kind of nightmares where he was booked in business class on a flight to Paris, but missed the taxi to the airport and tripped over and everything spilled out of his suitcase and someone stole something from him and he chased them down the street and someone else grabbed him and tied him up and threw him in a cupboard and he had to eat his way through a wooden door to get out. He put it down to stress.

His self-diagnosis was that he needed a holiday. He had a habit of taking on too many tasks at once: the pressures of recording the CD, designing the artwork, writing the program notes and planning the promotion were weighing on him. He owed money to relatives, friends and the bank. He was setting up a website to help young musicians launch their careers and, in his spare time, coaching a teenage cricket team. In some ways he was still a boy who loved to muck around, but he was also a generous and ambitious spirit, impatient to use his talents for a greater purpose.

Whatever was happening in his head had surprisingly little effect on his playing. Once Aaron had learned a piece of music, it was as if his hands rather than his brain remembered the notes. His long fingers skimmed across the keyboard. His legs, which had once carried him up and down basketball courts, never fitted under a piano, so he sat back, knees brushing the instrument, looking elegantly languid. Friends who dropped in to the studio heard only the resonant beauty of the music, never knowing that their presence distracted him so badly that he'd have to start again as soon as they were gone.

By July of 2001 he thought his head was going to explode. Still, he struggled on, promising himself that if he could just make it through the next few weeks he would go and lie on a beach.

Before making any holiday plans, however, he had to have some photographs taken for the album cover and, with absurdly bad timing, he developed an infection in his left eye. After a few days his eyelid was almost swollen shut and what he saw in the mirror was not photogenic.

That finally got his attention. Apart from the headaches, he was healthy, and it was years since he had seen a doctor. So he looked in the telephone book for a general practitioner close to the apartment he rented in a high-rise building in the oldest part of the city, The Rocks. There was a clinic just across Kent Street and as he walked in he noticed a sign on the receptionist's desk welcoming a new GP, Dr Barbara Schiff.

Barbara Schiff was a South African doctor who had just come through five years' study and training to requalify in Australia. Thursday 26 July was her first day in the practice and when Aaron turned up at 9 am, the brisk, blonde doctor was still unpacking. He liked to think he was her very first patient; he was certainly one of the first. He struck Schiff as a mature, personable young man who didn't want to be there. He was too busy.

'Something's wrong with my eye,' Aaron said.

He wasn't even going to mention the headaches. All he wanted was a quick treatment for the infection, a simple conjunctivitis. But Schiff hung on, questioning him about his medical history as she would with any new patient. Aaron found himself asking if he could have a blood test for diabetes. As a sugar addict who loved cakes and chocolates and baked a fine lemon meringue pie, he wondered if that might explain why he felt so low.

Eventually he mentioned his aching head and that prompted Schiff to dig a bit further. She was interested in her patients' overall wellbeing, and with young people, especially in big cities, she tried to get a psychological profile because depression and suicide were becoming so common. She also had an unusually expert knowledge of neurology. While waiting for a position in general practice, she had done postgraduate studies in rehabilitation and, as part of her training, had worked at Prince Henry Hospital in Sydney's Little Bay. Many of her patients had suffered spinal injuries, brain tumours, multiple sclerosis or strokes. When Aaron said 'headaches', she automatically began a series of tests on his vision.

'How many fingers am I holding up?' she asked, telling him to stare at her nose while she moved her hands quickly up and down, side to side, straight in front of him. Something wasn't quite right. She sent him away that day with a prescription for eye drops, a referral to Sydney Eye Hospital and an order to come back in four days.

Aaron bought the drops, his eye cleared up and he forgot both about visiting the eye hospital and seeing the doctor again. He was so close to finishing the CD. Four days after their first appointment his phone rang and, to his surprise, it was Schiff asking if he had been to the eye specialist and did he want to come in for that blood test.

As she drew blood from his arm the next day, she inquired about the headaches. Aaron described the pain as emanating from the centre of his head and causing pressure in his eyes. Maybe it was eyestrain, he said. After all, he had been staring at sheet music most of his life and wearing glasses since he was sixteen. She started on her tests again, checking his eyesight, reflexes, everything she could think of. Most of his reactions were normal – no loss of movement, no dilation of the pupils – until she held her fingers out in his lower left field of vision and asked what he could see.

'Is your hand still there?' he asked.

Schiff didn't show her concern but she wanted to know if he had vomited or been nauseous recently. As a matter of fact, just a few weeks before, he had been walking to the Sydney Cricket Ground for a coaching session and had had to sit down on a bench because he suddenly felt dizzy and sick. A bit further on, he had tripped over a chair at an outdoor cafe. Come to think of it, he'd been bumping into other low objects lately, as though he couldn't see them.

At the cricket ground he had bowled a few balls then collapsed. One of the boys, Elliot Bullock, shook him awake and Aaron had managed to stagger to the bathroom just before he vomited. Despite the violence of his attack, the nausea passed and he brushed it off as food poisoning or a virus.

'I don't want you to be alarmed but there's something going on here and you're going to have to have a CT scan,' said Schiff. 'I want you to go right now.'

Schiff still didn't allow herself to identify the problem but she got on the phone and made an appointment at an X-ray clinic in Macquarie Street. The words 'right now' echoed in Aaron's ears. An hour afterward, he lay under the scanner, still thinking about the music he would record later that day. The technician seemed uncomfortable as he said he'd send the scans to Schiff and that she would call him that evening.

Perhaps it wasn't a conscious decision, but instead of going straight home Aaron visited some neighbours. When he finally went up to his apartment the answering machine was blinking. Aaron pressed the button. Schiff's blunt South African voice said the news wasn't good and that she wanted to see him as soon as possible. In his mind, Aaron heard, 'brain tumour'.

He didn't know much about brain tumours, except that people died from them. There were no trivial thoughts about what time he was recording that night, or what music he should practise.

As he leaned back in his black executive chair, a mirror he had made at school seemed to shatter on the wall. He remembered later: 'You build up your life and work and things that mean something to you and suddenly the whole lot of them, everything around you, spins out. It's like it's not there anymore and the whole building and the desk and the chair and the piano fall away.'

When Aaron called Schiff ten minutes later, the questions poured out of him. What is it? How big is it? What does it mean? She didn't have the answers but told him lots of people got brain tumours and often they could be treated successfully.

'Take it a step at a time,' she said.

Aaron made two more phone calls that night. One was to Elliot, his fifteen-year-old cricketing friend, to warn him he wouldn't be up for coaching that week because he had a brain tumour, probably something about the size of a pea. Then he rang his grandparents, Frank and Marjorie Robinson, and told them he couldn't face the night alone.

'It will be all right, darling. Whatever it is, we'll deal with it,' said Marjorie.

*

Aaron was the first patient in Schiff's surgery next morning. Frank and Marjorie sat with him. Up on the light box, a series of scans showed an unmistakable cloudy white mass, a small explosion inside Aaron's head. It was much bigger than a pea – more like an orange.

Barbara Schiff had spent the previous night reading about brain tumours so that she could deal intelligently with the unusual situation. Most GPs have little experience of brain tumours and now she had to handle the consequences for Aaron and his family. She couldn't tell how large or deep the tumour was from the two-dimensional CT scans, and she had no idea what type it was, but she could see that its position towards the right rear of the brain made sense of the large blind spot she had discovered in Aaron's left peripheral vision.

Again she spoke urgently: 'You must go to hospital today.'

Prince Henry Hospital, where she had worked as a registrar, provided rehabilitation for patients from Prince of Wales Hospital at Randwick, in Sydney's east. She knew Prince of Wales had excellent neurology and neurosurgery departments, and one neurosurgeon had particularly impressed her. Although she had never met Charlie Teo, she had helped some of his patients. Occasionally she needed more information about a patient and she would contact his office. Unlike all the other consultants, who got their registrars to return the call, Charlie always spoke to her personally and she had learned a lot from listening to him. He seemed to regard his patients as people rather than just cases.

Charlie Teo was the man she wanted. But he worked mainly at Prince of Wales Private Hospital and Aaron had no health insurance – what 24-year-old thinks he's going to need major surgery? – and no money for expensive private care. Taking in Charlie's fee of two and a half to five thousand dollars, hospital and operation fees, medications, X-rays and so on, costs usually amounted to about twenty-five thousand dollars, and with complications could reach fifty thousand. So she could only send him to the public wing. There were no guarantees that Charlie would see him. She told Aaron to go to Emergency and rang the hospital to say he was on his way.

Aaron arrived at the hospital with his grandparents, his scans and no idea what was going to happen. He gave his details to the triage nurse at the reception desk and stepped away.

A woman behind the desk flipped through his scans and asked her colleagues too loudly, 'When did this one die?'

'No, no,' one of them said quickly. 'He's just come in.'

Even so, his wasn't the most urgent case. There was a long wait before they were taken up a corridor to a tiny room, bare except for a bed. Eventually a registrar came to say that the neurosurgeon was operating and might not be free for five hours. Aaron decided it wasn't fair to keep his grandparents there so he sent them home, got some food from a vending machine, sat on the bed and rang his mate Elliot.

'It ain't a pea.'

2

HOLY SHIT

A cluster of medical students leaned in as Charlie Teo held up Aaron's CT scans for the first time.

'Holy shit!' he said in his broad Australian accent. 'Look at that . . . Look at that bit.'

Even though he had operated on some four thousand brain tumours, this one was big, it was in a dangerous area, and its cauliflower-shaped outline looked like nothing he'd seen before. 'Deadly' was the word that came to mind. Charlie Teo the surgeon had an almighty challenge ahead but Charlie Teo the showman and teacher also had an opportunity for some theatre in front of the students.

A young registrar named Ralph Mobbs had been the first to assess Aaron when he was admitted on Wednesday 1 August. He noted in the records that the patient was a musician ('piano player – apparently v. famous') and that he was 'alert, oriented and v. worried!' Aaron had told him he felt 'lethargic' and 'stressed out', that he had suffered from early-morning headaches and one vomiting episode and had been walking into furniture and door-frames on his left side. Otherwise, he was 'in good health'. His CT scans showed a lesion measuring six by six centimetres in the right occipital lobe, the area at the back of the brain that processes visual information and recognises shapes and colours.

Neurosurgeons at Prince of Wales take it in turns to handle the urgent head injuries, strokes, tumours and other central nervous system cases that come in through Emergency. After looking at Aaron's scans, Ralph Mobbs had contacted Charlie, who was becoming well known for taking on tumours other surgeons considered inoperable.

Charlie was operating on a private patient but, as soon as he had a break, he went next door to the public hospital. Aaron could hear a ripple of excitement long before the doctor and his entourage appeared in his holding cell. He had only been waiting a couple of hours but word seemed to have got around that he was an unusual case. He heard Charlie's 'Holy shit!' from the corridor.

Doctor and patient were both surprised by what they saw. Aaron had overheard nurses on the ward talking about the amazing, talented Dr Teo, but the hotshot surgeon he was expecting looked no older than the students squeezing in behind him. Aaron thought of Doogie Howser, the teenage doctor in the 1980s US television series. Surely he was no more than thirty, this slender man with Chinese features, shorn black hair and a direct manner.

'You're Aaron, are you?' Charlie said, taking in the tall, blond and unexpectedly healthy-looking young man on the bed. He was wary after being told this guy was a bit of a VIP, a pianist who had made albums and toured the world. People often tried to big-note themselves to get special treatment and Charlie refused to fall for that. If this guy was so famous, why was he a public patient?

When Aaron told the story of how he came to hospital that day, Charlie was impressed that Barbara Schiff had correctly suspected a brain tumour. Patients with worse symptoms could go for months or years, seeing doctor after doctor, before they found out what was wrong. If she hadn't been so acute, Aaron might have died from another seizure like his attack on the cricket field.

Charlie taught his students to assess a patient's appearance before looking at their scans or other test results. With Aaron, there was little to see: he moved and talked normally and seemed very self-possessed. Yet, the CT scans showed a growth filling a quarter of his head.

Charlie turned from the scans back to Aaron and said, 'I'm not sure what type of tumour this is but it looks like a very, very serious one and it's going to have to come out. We're going to operate. I want you to go home and get your things and we'll admit you to the ward today. Then we'll just take it from there.'

'How long is this going to take?' Aaron asked. 'Are we talking a week? I've got to finish recording an album.'

Charlie had never heard anyone react so coolly. Most patients cried or just stopped listening at that point. Most also had a relative or friend present to hold them together. 'You little upstart,' he thought. 'I've just told you you have a brain tumour and you want to finish an album?'

'Hang on, Aaron. Get your priorities straight. I don't think you quite understand what I'm saying. This tumour is about to kill you. If we don't operate, you probably have about six weeks to live. We're not talking about finishing an album. We're talking about trying to save your life.'

This time Aaron understood. The last threads of connection with his old life snapped. He muttered something: yes, yes, whatever you think. There was talk of drugs and costs, and softer words about looking after him, but all he heard was, 'Six weeks . . .'

Aaron rang his grandparents, then walked back through the noisy triage area, where other emergencies had overtaken his, and out the glass front doors. A cold wind swirled up the driveway, and a stream of ambulances and family cars delivered new patients. Soon a heavy rain began to fall and Aaron stood under it. If he was going to die, why worry about getting wet? Unaware of his crisis, Frank and Marjorie finished their chores and it was three hours before their car pulled in at the hospital. Aaron fell onto the back seat, a drenched, sobbing mess.

At his apartment, he packed a suitcase. He had only recently moved in and the place was barely furnished, but it seemed as if he were leaving a familiar nest.

There was no bed available in the wards when they got back to the hospital, so Aaron returned to the tiny room where he had spent most of the day. Sitting with his grandparents, slightly calmer, he began to think about who needed to know what was happening. He'd thought he would tell almost no one, not even his mother. He would just say he was going on a trip and disappear for a month, the way people do when they have a face-lift. He could avoid hurting anyone, and it would all be less of a drama. But the plan was starting to seem ridiculous.

His mother, Gail Puckett, had moved to Brisbane the previous year and was sorting out her life there with Aaron's stepfather and their two children. When Aaron was a child it had been just the two of them muddling through on love and instinct, and their ties were strong, if slightly frayed. Aaron sent his grandparents – Gail's parents – out of the room and rang her.

'Something really bad has happened. I've been diagnosed with a brain tumour the size of an orange and I've got six weeks to live.'

Aaron thought the words would knock her out but she reacted just as he had. 'I'll have to come down,' she said and started planning aloud when she could get away from the Rudolf Steiner school where she taught, maybe sometime the following week. Gradually the news sank in and when Marjorie came in and took the phone, both women were choked with tears.

Late that night, Aaron was moved upstairs to the neurosurgery unit in Ward 8. The nurse who admitted him took note of a 'well-dress[ed] and young male, looked depress[ed] . . . cooperative and anxious'.

It was an odd time to be there. Prince of Wales was built in the 1960s and, apart from a few coats of the washed-out pastel paints common to hospitals, there had been no refurbishment of the wards in almost forty years. As their physical condition deteriorated, so had the staff's morale. When Aaron arrived, the nursing unit manager, Ashley Eastwood, had ten job vacancies she couldn't fill and was getting by with pool and agency nurses to help her overworked staff. Meanwhile, renovations were finally about to begin so the neurology patients had been moved out, leaving only neurosurgery. Half the floor was shut down and deserted.

Aaron's world shrank to his room and, behind a pink curtain, a man in the other bed who was friendly enough between bouts of diarrhoea. Aaron tried to concentrate on who he had to contact. As he rang some people, they rang others and word flew that the shining young pianist had been struck down. At the same time he was adjusting to being a patient. Apart from his headache he still didn't feel like a sick person, but the hospital had to keep him alive until surgery.

Erica Jacobsen was the neurosurgery registrar put in charge of the tests and treatments and plans for Aaron's operation. A bright young woman with short red hair and a ready laugh, she would be one of only nine female neurosurgeons in Australia when she went into practice two years later. She had studied piano at the Sydney Conservatorium of Music as a child, and she liked Aaron and appreciated his talent.

She knew the diagnosis of a brain tumour could be overwhelming, but Aaron was frank and friendly and wanted straight answers. He told Jacobsen and the staff what he needed; they told him what they had to do.

Aaron was put on dexamethasone, a steroid which would reduce the swelling in his brain and lessen the chance of another seizure. The feeling of pressure, as though his head were being squeezed, subsided. His field of vision was tested more scientifically, by an examiner, who flashed spots of light onto a large screen and asked Aaron to respond when he saw them. Half the time, Aaron was silent. His printed test results showed two circles, representing each eye, densely sprinkled with dots where his vision was normal. The left half of both circles was blank.

Eyesight follows a complicated path. At first, the left optic nerve carries visual information into the brain from the entire left eye and the right optic nerve from the right eye. But, at a certain point, the nerves cross and swap part of their bundles. The nerve that travels on to the left occipital lobe takes information from the right visual field of both eyes, while the other takes information from the left half of both eyes to the right occipital lobe. The flow of images through Aaron's brain was interrupted by pressure from the tumour on that final destination point.

He hadn't noticed his narrowing eyesight because of another brain skill. Everyone has a small blind spot at the point where the optic nerve leaves the eye and the retina has no light-sensitive neurons. Most of the time there's no hole in our vision because each eye sees what the other misses. But, more than that, the brain can fill in blind spots by imagining what it expects to see – and usually gets it right.

Aaron had been tripping and bumping into objects on his left side without realising that he couldn't see them. He compensated with a combination of 'filling in' and turning his head so that the right side of his visual field took over. But even if the bass end of his piano keyboard had disappeared from view, his piano playing was more about memory and touch than sight. And yet the tumour was very close to the adjoining parietal lobe, which controls spatial sense, the ability to move around and reach for objects. On the right side of the brain it also controls artistic expression. Somehow, despite the other interruptions to his brain function, his musical dexterity survived. Perhaps he was adapted to overcome such an intrusion. The brains of professional musicians have recently been found to have more grey matter than amateur and non-musicians in the three areas dealing with motor skills, auditory stimulation, and visual and spatial data. Whether the difference is genetic or built up over years of practice is not certain, though it appears that the younger a child takes up music, the greater the development in the auditory cortex. As the British neurologist Oliver Sacks writes in *Musicophilia*, 'Anatomists today would be hard put to identify the brain of a visual artist, a writer, or a mathematician – but they could recognise the brain of a professional musician without a moment's hesitation.'

Erica Jacobsen believed that Aaron's brain was wired differently because he had been a pianist since childhood, and that this had helped him function despite the tumour. Still, she wondered how he was using his left hand and playing as well as he did.

Magnetic resonance imaging scans, known as MRIs, gave a more detailed anatomical view inside Aaron's head. Against the dark grey of his brain, the tumour stood out like a puff of white cumulus cloud. It looked insubstantial, almost innocent.

More than a hundred varieties of tumour can strike the central nervous system in a multitude of forms: neat eggs; dark, splotchy stains; jelly-like deposits; pale, rubbery inserts that adapt their shape to fill the spaces in the brain called ventricles; bubbly bunches of grapes; or coral-shaped growths. The incidence of brain cancer had risen inexplicably around the world in the past decade from the fifteenth to the ninth most common cancer in adults and, after leukaemia, the most common in children. The most lethal forms are also the most frequent.

But Aaron's tumour didn't look to Charlie like a highly malignant astrocytoma. Nor did it look like a common and relatively benign meningioma, which grows from the membrane covering the brain. He tossed around the possibilities with his registrars and other neurosurgeons, and at a radiology meeting and his Tuesday morning tutorial with the medical students.

Erica Jacobsen was working towards her exams and had a head full of information. She noted that the tumour was unusually large and seemed to be growing from the falx, a part of the membrane that forms a partition down the middle of the brain. She also considered the fact that Aaron was a young male. Based on these three details, at one of the neurosurgeons' meetings she took an intelligent guess.

'Could it be a hemangiopericytoma?'

Charlie jumped on the idea. 'Shit. I think that's exactly what it is.'

Nothing could be confirmed until the tumour was put under a microscope and tested by pathology, but Erica had hit on a rare type that Charlie had seen no more than half a dozen times in his career. They make up less than one per cent of all primary nervous system tumours. They originate in the covering membrane rather than the brain tissue itself, yet are classed as malignant because they grow fast and have a high rate of re-currence. As the name suggests, they are fed by a network of blood vessels. Most often they occur in young men. Like all brain tumours, their cause is a mystery.

Aaron was young and clean-living – he never smoked, barely drank, didn't own a mobile phone; sugar and overwork were his only vices. What genetic seed had been planted in him? What invisible poison had touched him? Or what unjust finger of fate?

3

UTOPIA

While Aaron faced what might be the last six weeks of his life, Charlie was searching for a way to avoid operating on him. For starters, he hated working in the public health system. 'I wouldn't send my dog to a public hospital,' he said to patients, doctors, journalists, anyone he could. 'I would only send my worst enemy. The equipment's not as good; the staffing isn't as good; you have no team spirit; it's a can't-do mentality. It's not even a factory because a factory tries to get people through as quickly as it can. The public system doesn't want people. If they could, they'd have an empty hospital because that's the least cost to them.'

Public hospitals don't suit Charlie's personality, or his modus operandi. In his private practice he has built an intimate team around him, from anaesthetists to registrars and receptionists. He trains three or four nurses to work in theatres with him, so they are familiar with his personalised instruments, know how to hand them to him, and enjoy – or at least tolerate – his jokes and his musical taste. He gives credit to his team when an operation goes well and often takes them out to dinner or back to his house for a party. In return, they give him unshakable loyalty. But even he admits he can be demanding. When Kate Joseph joined his nursing team, he told her, 'I'm perfect and I expect you to be perfect too.'

Prince of Wales is a teaching hospital, a sprawling campus of late-twentieth-century buildings attached to the neighbouring University of New South Wales. As well as their main responsibility to patients, the public and children's hospitals are obliged to offer hands-on experience to trainee doctors.

Charlie loves teaching, invites students to watch him operate and bonds closely with most of his registrars. But he is edgy when he operates in the public hospital, as he doesn't always have his own instruments and many of the staff are strangers. He wonders whether the anaesthetist is replacing lost blood and accurately monitoring the patient's vital signs. He has to look up when a new nurse gives him the wrong scissors. He has to watch his manners. Sometimes he even has to turn down the volume on John Denver to stop people shouting at him.

His reluctance to perform Aaron's high-risk operation under these conditions was increased by his professional history. It was only two years since Charlie had returned to Sydney from the United States, where he had trained and practised for almost a decade in Texas and Arkansas. A few Australian neurosurgeons had not welcomed him back.

Among the small, conservative neurosurgical community – just over a hundred in Australia and New Zealand, and about thirty of them in New South Wales, concentrated in Sydney – Charlie Teo is regarded by many as an eccentric. He runs, he cycles, he has a black belt in karate, he kayaks around Sydney Harbour and he plays the bagpipes dressed in a kilt. To ensure he has an iron-steady operating hand, he does not drink alcohol or caffeine. Under the operating microscope he can see a colleague's hand shake after just one cup of coffee – lethal if you're cutting into human flesh. Then he sweeps aside all his cautious habits by riding to work on a motorbike, most recently a black Honda 900RR Fireblade – the kind of sexy machine that is responsible for many of the head trauma cases he treats every year. He loves speed and what he calls 'manageable risk'. He had three accidents in the early days and broke a thumb and damaged a knee. The worst, when he was an intern, landed him in jail overnight for punching a driver who had run him and his girlfriend off the road, knocking them from their bike and leaving the girl bloody and unconscious.

Charlie is outspoken, ebullient, informal in his dress and bedside manner. His humour often comes from another age, both adolescent and pre-feminist. He flirts with nurses and, though he does not mean to offend, occasionally goes too far with his hugs and teasing and dirty jokes. He is boastful in a specialty full of large egos that are usually not on public display. Many of them talk about neurosurgery as a club that only admits members with the right image, or a psychiatric ward where dozens of Jesus Christs stand around arguing with each other – and then in walks Charlie Teo and says, 'Yes, but *I'm* the Messiah.'

Most neurosurgeons refuse to speak to the media. Apart from the tacit rules of the profession against publicity and competition, they consider it to be in bad taste. Charlie, on the other hand, gave his first interview in 1988, when he was still in training. The story in *The Sun Herald* began: 'Dr Charlie Teo has the reputation of being the hardest working registrar at Sydney's Royal Prince Alfred Hospital.' The superlative was probably true. Thirty-year-old Charlie worked a hundred hours a week and thirteen days a fortnight, operating for at least eight hours a day before ward duties and evening call, reluctant to claim overtime and rarely seeing his fiancée. He never took holidays and claimed his only sick day after blistering his bare feet on hot bitumen while he helped push a stranger's broken-down car. He couldn't have been happier with the workload.

'It's a great thrill to save someone's life. I save a life probably once a week . . . I want people to know I'm working my backside off,' he told the newspaper.

New South Wales doctors were on strike over their long working hours and the journalist's intention was to back up their claims. Charlie's colleagues had recommended him for the interview; one said he would have worked twenty-six hours in a twenty-four-hour day if it were possible. Charlie warned the reporter that he was really the wrong guy to speak to because he *liked* working long hours; he wanted to soak up as much experience as possible.

On the day the story appeared, he was fired from the hospital. The board of the Neurosurgical Society of Australasia wanted to know why he was appearing as a pin-up boy for the strike. It took a letter of apology from Charlie, a statutory declaration from the journalist and a promise not to speak to the media anymore to save him. But he was marked.

A short time later, he was fired again. He was at work at six o'clock one morning when a patient fell out of bed and developed a dangerous blood clot in his head. The chairman of the department was the patient's neurosurgeon but he was still on his way to the hospital, so Charlie broke the rules. He left the chairman a message that he was doing the operation himself. At that moment, saving a life seemed more important than the strict protocol of not touching another doctor's patient.

The operation went well but when Charlie emerged from the theatre he was called to the office of the clinical superintendent, who said the chairman wanted him fired on the spot. Charlie cried. It looked as though his career was at an end. His mentor, Ian Johnston, associate professor of neurosurgery at the University of Sydney and a leading neurosurgeon at the hospital, intervened, and the other registrars and residents signed petitions in Charlie's support. After three days of hell he was reinstated.

Charlie failed his final exam in neurosurgery twice. Failure is not uncommon in such a demanding specialty. But when his results came back the second time, he asked his supervisor where he had gone wrong.

'I need to talk to you about that,' said the supervisor, sitting down on his desk and taking off his glasses. The problem was nothing to do with Charlie's ability as a surgeon; it was his attitude and his image. Whether he liked it or not, society put neurosurgeons on a pedestal and expected them to behave with dignity and authority.

'What do you want me to do, change my personality?' asked Charlie.

No, said the older man; he should just change three things: stop calling patients by their first names and letting them use his first name; stop nightclubbing and settle down; and get rid of the motorbike!

In January 1989 Charlie married Genevieve Agnew, taking a long weekend off work for their honeymoon. He had pursued the Perth-born beauty for three years after meeting her at Concord Hospital, where she was a nurse and he was a resident. As well as settling down, he stopped calling patients by their first names and quit riding his motorbike – at least until he passed his exam on the third attempt.

To celebrate his victory, another neurosurgeon, Steve Halcrow, gave him a present – a pair of grey socks with the words *World's greatest fuck* written in a red patch on the sides. As well as liking the joke, and maybe believing it, Charlie was touched. Steve was an eccentric too: straggly-haired, unshaven and frequently mumbling. After leaving Australia to train in Belfast he had had trouble breaking into the system back in Sydney. But Charlie saw the clever, careful surgeon behind the idiosyncracies and helped him get a job. The two men would remain friends and allies long after their careers took them to different parts of the world. Charlie insisted on wearing his lucky socks during every difficult operation for more than a decade, until they were in shreds. A neurosurgeon had to believe he was a superhero just to keep going and those socks helped him feel like a winner.

After twelve years of education and training, Charlie wasn't even sure he'd be given a job in Australia. Besides, he wanted to be a paediatric neurosurgeon and believed the most advanced and exciting work in the field was being done in the United States. Ian Johnston wanted to offer him a research fellowship or organise a year of overseas experience. But Charlie did it the hard way. He picked the best chapters from the latest American textbook on paediatric neurosurgery and wrote to the authors asking for a job. With half a dozen replies in hand, he flew to America for interviews and landed a fellowship at the Children's Medical Center in Dallas, Texas.

In 1991 he and Genevieve, his wife of almost three years, left the fibro house in Balmain that he had renovated for the wealthy suburbs of Dallas. He worked with three paediatric neurosurgeons, who gave him a broad perspective. He was impressed by the American can-do attitude and they were impressed by his skills and hard work. The children on the wards were thrilled at Halloween to see a Chinese man with an Australian accent in a kilt playing the bagpipes; he became a hospital legend. By the time he was thinking of heading home a year later, job offers were coming from all over the States. From Australia, neurosurgeons told him he would do well there and should stay. Their encouragement was also a warning, which he took. He restudied basic medicine, sat for the exams and became the only medical board–certified Australian neurosurgeon in America. One of his referees was Ed Laws, the president of the American Association of Neurosurgeons, who told him the chief of paediatric neurosurgery at Arkansas Children's Hospital was retiring and they would like him to apply for the position.

Little Rock, Arkansas, was home of the former governor and newly elected president, Bill Clinton. The Children's Hospital was well funded, thanks to support from Hillary Clinton, and had one of the best neurosurgery units in the States, built up by its visionary chairman, Ossama Al-Mefty.

When the faculty told Charlie the job was his, he turned it down. For Genevieve, already far from home and nursing their first baby, Little Rock seemed like a Bible-Belt backwater. But the hospital wooed them hard and in 1994 Charlie was appointed assistant professor of neurosurgery at the University of Arkansas for Medical Sciences, vice-chief of paediatric neurosurgery at the Children's Hospital and acting chief of neurosurgery at John L McClellan Memorial Veterans Hospital in Little Rock.

He was in surgical heaven. Within six weeks he had set up a multidisciplinary clinic specialising in brain tumours, with

its own building, nurses, advertising and state-of-the-art endoscopic equipment.

Endoscopy was Charlie's ace in the hole. He had learned
the technique at Prince of Wales Hospital, where he used a tiny,
powerful microscope that could be inserted on a long cable
into bodily cavities such as the abdomen, the nasal sinuses and
the ventricles in the brain. The endoscope turned corners, illu-
minated dark spots and allowed the surgeon to work through
a small incision.

Bernard Kwok, Bob Jones and Warwick Stening, all senior
neurosurgeons at Prince of Wales, had begun using endoscopy
in the late 1970s to treat certain types of hydrocephalus, the
build-up of spinal fluid on the brain. Instead of doing it the old
way, placing a piece of tubing called a shunt under the skin
to drain excess fluid, they performed a simple operation to bypass
the blocked passages and create a hole in the base of the ventricle.

Charlie took the technique to the States, where it was hardly
known. Other doctors noted that his patients usually left hospital
a day after surgery and recovered surprisingly well. He was sure
that such an effective technique would have many applications.
Pituitary tumours had been removed through the nostril for
decades but surgeons had to make an incision under the lip
and lift up the nose. It took half an hour just to get in there and
the surgery was painful and destructive. Charlie worked out how
to insert the endoscope up the nostril in a procedure taking five
minutes.

He was soon travelling and teaching and taking referrals
from around the world. He progressed to associate professor of
neurosurgery at the University of Arkansas and chief of paediatric
neurosurgery at Arkansas Children's Hospital, whose department had expanded from four to fourteen neurosurgeons,

making it the third largest in North America. Most of Charlie's operations were on children but he also developed a reputation for taking on difficult adult tumours that other surgeons didn't want to touch.

When he presented his results at a meeting, someone would invariably compliment him and ask if they could watch him operate. The only notable country that didn't invite him to conferences was Australia. Finally he decided to visit anyway.

At the 1998 meeting of the International Society of Pediatric Neurosurgeons in Melbourne, Charlie presented his results in the endoscopic removal of third-ventricular brain tumours, a difficult operation that had a mortality of about sixty per cent and a morbidity of one hundred per cent. In other words, no one came out fully functioning. Charlie gave the results for thirty-nine patients he had operated on using the endoscope: all had survived without complications or long-term deficit. His mother, Elizabeth Teo, was in the audience and heard people sniggering as her son spoke. Not a single person thanked Charlie after his talk. No one believed him.

By contrast, Charlie thrived in the bigger, less conservative and highly competitive American neurosurgical community. Even his admirers would occasionally shake their heads and ask, 'What's he up to now?' but he was widely liked, respected as a pioneering surgeon and teacher and, most of the time, allowed to be himself.

One incident, however, threatened to derail him. A senior nurse at Arkansas Children's Hospital filed a sexual harassment complaint in 1996 after seeing him sit close to a younger nurse and ask if she was married. Charlie thought he was just showing his usual brash friendliness, and was horrified to think he had caused offence. He wrote the young nurse a letter of apology. She rang, confused. She had made no complaint. She had never found his behaviour inappropriate and told him there was no need to apologise. Charlie hired a lawyer and the hospital dismissed the complaint. But the incident was wiped from his record only after he got letters of support from a senator and an oil magnate who were his patients, and from Bill Clinton's personal physician.

Charlie was working a hundred hours a week in his utopia. In almost nine years in America he reckoned he had operated on more than five hundred new paediatric brain tumours, five times as much experience as he would have got at an Australian hospital. He loved camping and canoeing in the Ozark Mountains and driving his red Ferrari. At home in their hundred-year-old, white-pillared house, however, Genevieve had three little girls and was pregnant with a fourth. She missed Australia.

The final straw came when Alexandra, their eldest, had gunfire drill at school. Massacres in US schools were becoming unnervingly commonplace. One of four shootings in 1998 occurred near Jonesboro, Arkansas, where two boys, aged thirteen and eleven, shot dead four other students and a teacher and wounded ten more. At Alex's school that year, the children were taught that if they heard gunfire they must drop to the floor, combat crawl towards the teacher and leave the room in single file, helping injured classmates if they could.

Charlie had achieved more in his years in the US than he had ever dreamed he would, but decided that Australia would be better for his family if not his career. As they were getting ready to leave, the University of California, San Diego offered him the position of chairman of paediatric neurosurgery. At forty-two, he would have been one of the youngest chairmen in the country, and he was tempted. A senior neurosurgeon there, who had been a visiting professor in Australia, warned, 'Charlie, you're not going to be happy in Australia. You're going to be wishing you accepted this job.' Undaunted, the Teo family packed their belongings and prepared to move back home.

4

HOME ALONE

If Aaron was busy before his diagnosis, now he had hardly a moment to himself.

He quickly realised what it meant to be in a teaching hospital: he was a specimen. Every day groups of doctors and students trooped into his room to examine him. One morning a nurse rushed in with a wheelchair and said, 'Come on, you have to go for your tests.' She grabbed his scans from the files in the corridor, wheeled him out to the lifts and into a room full of students. The supervising professor explained to Aaron that the students in this room would try to diagnose his illness from a physical examination, while a group in another room would look at his scans and describe what condition they expected the patient to be in.

For the next couple of hours the students filed in two by two. They got him to stick out his tongue, asked questions to test his memory, and noted he could move his eyes easily. They did eyesight tests with their fingers but not one picked up the gap in his peripheral vision. No one asked about vomiting. Aaron played games with them; when a student tapped his skin to check his sense of touch, he would fling out his arm. The student looked disconcerted until Aaron and the others started giggling. When they looked at his scans they were stunned. No one had guessed he had a brain tumour.

When he walked into the next room, a chorus of 'Wow!' rose from the students who had been looking at his scans. Six had decided he would be in a coma by now and four had said he should be dead. They learned that the most diligent study could not always explain real human beings.

There was no nurse or wheelchair to take Aaron back to his bed, so he wandered around until he found his way back to the ward on level 8. 'Where on earth have you been?' asked a nurse. It turned out that the morning tests had been 'unofficial', one more sign of the growing interest in his case around the hospital. Aaron felt the students were treating him as if he were a quiz question: Guess what's wrong with this guy? Can you work it out? The nurses were briefed to stop intruders from wandering in.

Visitors began to arrive, initially just a trickle. Among the first were Steve Leong and Andi Gabereder, two young men who lived in Aaron's apartment building. Aaron had become like a brother to them. He helped Steve with his piano playing; Andi cooked dinner; and they often talked into the morning after Aaron came home from his recording sessions, exhausted and sleepless. Only a week before, he had complained about his head-aches, squeezing Steve's scalp and saying, 'It feels like this.'

He had rung the pair from the hospital in the darkest hours of the night and said, 'I don't want to die.' Steve and Andi cancelled their upcoming holiday in New Caledonia and, as others would, planned to help Aaron as much as possible. At the hospital the next day, he hugged them and joked with the nurses but they could see the lonely, frightened boy behind the performance.

Another early visitor to the hospital was Aaron's father, Brian McMillan. Brian felt that he owed a debt to his son and here was an opportunity to repay some of it. Even before Aaron was born, Brian had run away from the responsibility of fatherhood, ending up in Thailand, where he spent eight years as a Buddhist monk and several more caught up with drugs. Since reappearing in Sydney when Aaron was seventeen, he had gradually, sometimes clumsily, worked at being a father.

Aaron's mother, Gail Puckett, arrived from Brisbane with her daughter, Amy, having taken indefinite leave from her job. Aaron could see the pain on his mother's face as she contemplated losing her son, as well as the strain of facing Brian again after so many years.

Peter Crisp made the four-hour drive from his family property at Yass, where he worked as a glass artist and held concerts in a corrugated-iron shed. Aaron had played there and they shared what Peter called the 'universal consciousness' of artists. At the hospital he became a quiet, practical fixture, taking phone calls and shepherding the crowds.

More than forty visitors passed through Aaron's room over that first weekend. Often he came back from a test to find a friend sitting in the chair and four more on his bed. The nurses noted, occasionally with disapproval, that his visitors stayed as late as midnight, long after visiting hours.

Simon Creedy, a graphic designer who had been working on Aaron's website and album-in-progress, turned up to see him emerge dazed from having MRI scans. He made Aaron laugh, as he always did, babbling about how he'd saved money by parking illegally in a lane inside the hospital grounds. He spirited Aaron out of the hospital to go for a drive in his new fat-tyred car and buy ice-cream at the beach.

Aaron was an enigma, even to his intimates, a textbook Aquarian who could have been the model for Linda Goodman's description in her astrology classic, *Sun Signs*, which begins: 'Lots of people like rainbows . . . but the Aquarian is ahead of everybody. He lives on one. What's more, he's taken it apart and examined it, piece by piece, colour by colour, and he still believes in it.' His mother and stepfather characterised him as the *puer aeternus*, the eternal youth of Greek mythology and Jungian psychology, while Peter Pan and Antoine de Saint-Exupéry's Little Prince were the literary embodiments of the archetype. Creative and optimistic, they saw life as a grand quest but sometimes had difficulty with real-life commitments to jobs, people and responsibility. Some of them died young, perhaps because they couldn't imagine growing old. But it seemed that Aaron's not-quite-here quality was also his protection from the trials of his body.

Charlie came to see Aaron with his mother and grandparents soon after Gail's arrival. Again, he spoke plainly. Usually he told patients they had less than one per cent risk of dying during surgery, but because of the size and location of Aaron's tumour, his risk of death was as high as five to ten per cent (later he would tell Gail that her son's chance of survival was even worse than he had let on to Aaron) and there was no chance that he would survive without some sort of damage. But there was also no choice. The time bomb ticking in Aaron's head could go off any day. And so far, Charlie had not lost a patient on the operating table.

Talking about the organ he had studied for twenty years, Charlie said, 'We've only touched the tip of the iceberg. Just the basic physiology of spinal fluid, for example, is still a mystery. I mean, why do we have spinal fluid? Some people say you need it to cushion the brain, it's got to swim in this water. But woodpeckers don't have spinal fluid around their brains and if anyone needs their brain to be cushioned it's bloody woodpeckers.'

Spinal fluid does play a role in making the human brain so resilient and adaptable that it can ignore an invader the size of an orange for months or even years. Every time a person sneezes or stands on his head, blood rushes to the brain. Instead of being crushed inside the skull, the brain compensates for its momentary expansion by shooting a few drops of spinal fluid out into the spinal column to make extra space. This tiny balancing act happens thousands of times a day, like so many other silent, involuntary biological functions. But the brain is also as fragile as an egg. A tumour like Aaron's caused pressure and swelling as it grew. For a long time the brain compensated as usual but eventually the balancing mechanisms broke down. All the spinal fluid had been pushed out and there was still no space. Aaron's brain was under such pressure when he arrived at the hospital that a simple cough could have caused a massive rise in pressure, brain herniation, a seizure – even death.

His operation should have been scheduled for the week after he was admitted. However, there was an impediment. His tumour was not only large but very vascular, stealing blood from the brain though a network of large and tiny vessels. Cutting into them would cause copious and possibly fatal bleeding. Charlie wanted to send Aaron to another specialist for a procedure called embolisation, which would close off some of the blood vessels to the tumour, making the surgeon's job easier. Charlie wanted

Dr Geoffrey Parker, a neuroradiologist at Royal Prince Alfred Hospital, to perform Aaron's embolisation. However, Parker was skiing in Thredbo. Charlie decided it wouldn't hurt Aaron to wait and that he could go home for a week.

The nurse's record for Monday 6 August notes that Aaron was 'awake and wandering the ward long into night'. But compared with most of the patients that Ashley Eastwood cared for on the ward, he seemed like a strapping, spirited young man. He was often walking around and chatting with his friends. With a queue of sicker patients always waiting for a hospital bed, anyone who could manage alone was sent home.

On Tuesday 7 August, Aaron was discharged. Gail planned to stay with him and make sure he took his pills, but he was irritable and sent her away. He felt vulnerable and, after staring over the precipice at emergency surgery and an unknown future, being back at home seemed anticlimactic. He crossed the street to tell Barbara Schiff, the GP, how grateful he was that she had diagnosed him correctly. Mostly he lay on his mattress while the visitors and phone calls kept coming. Two of his teenage cricket stars, Nick and Jason, arrived in a state of anxiety. Aaron tried to explain his illness and his treatment as they held on to him as if he might disappear.

Early that evening, he began to feel nauseous and faint, very much as he'd felt before his first seizure. Andi was at home when Aaron's weak voice came on the phone saying he had to go to hospital. Upstairs Andi found Aaron grey and crying, fumbling with his pills and near collapse. Barbara Schiff ordered an ambulance for the trip back to Prince of Wales.

Aaron arrived at Emergency on a gurney, barely a week after he had first walked in. He had to go through the long admissions process again. Andi and Steve were terrified, as he seemed to be losing consciousness. They left a message for Gail and, late that night, after catching a train, a bus and a taxi from her parents' house, she ran through the doors, equally distraught.

Squeezed in with all the other emergency patients on wheels, like dodgem cars, Aaron felt for the first time that he would like to slip away from the pain and the drips and the moaning around him. He was drifting into blackness when he heard someone say they had found him a bed. He clung on until he heard Gail's voice: 'I'm here.'

5

THE COWBOY

Back in Sydney after nine years in the US, Charlie and Genevieve Teo moved into a comfortable Federation house in Sydney's eastern suburbs and enrolled their girls in a local public school. Charlie was ready to settle down. Despite what he said about public hospitals, he was determined to get an academic job that would place him at the centre of the government system. Not only was he keen to keep teaching, he wanted to improve the patients' chances in the lottery of public hospital care.

He applied for positions as a paediatric neurosurgeon at two hospitals. One job, created by his old mentor Ian Johnston with Charlie in mind, was withdrawn when there were no other applicants. Another went to a candidate without any paediatric experience. He then applied unsuccessfully for an associate professorship in neurosurgery at the University of New South Wales and Prince of Wales Hospital but the job went instead to

Marcus Stoodley, a decade less experienced than Charlie and cut from a different cloth. Built like a rugby player, softly spoken, friendly but not effusive, Stoodley had spent years in a research laboratory to get his PhD in neurovascular surgery. An academic job requires the ability to run a lab and he had the advantage there. Perhaps it also had something to do with the fact that he could, years later, proudly show me his personal contacts list and say, 'Look, I do not have Channel Nine's phone number.' Charlie did, of course, and Stoodley disapproved of his close relationship with the media.

In spite of their differences, the two men respected each other. But Charlie believed he had been blocked from all those jobs for no better reason than political opposition from neurosurgeons who disliked him. His wife thought he was still seen as the wild registrar he had been a decade earlier. There were even whispers that he had left America because of the false harassment story. But Bernard Kwok, the chairman of neurosurgery at Prince of Wales, championed him, and another neurosurgeon who had worked closely with Charlie argued that there was something wrong with the prejudice against him.

A member of one selection committee asked Charlie if he was a team player. Yes, he said. He had a multidisciplinary clinic in Little Rock with eight specialists and everyone got on well.

But what if he weren't in charge of the clinic?

'I would still be a team player,' he said without hesitation.

That wasn't the truth. Charlie knew he was only a team player when he was the captain; he was a strong leader and a lousy follower.

With no academic job forthcoming, he set up in private practice, based at Prince of Wales Private Hospital, and as a consultant to the public and children's hospitals. His focus remained on children's tumours and especially on cases that other doctors judged to be inoperable. He set up the Centre for Minimally Invasive Neurosurgery, a clinic and training ground for the advanced techniques he applied with such encouraging results: small incisions and keyhole craniotomies, neuroendoscopy, reduced trauma to the brain and fast recovery. He established a comfortable rhythm to his week. On Monday and Wednesday he operated on private patients, often long into the night; on Tuesday he saw patients in his rooms; on Thursday he was in the public operating theatres; and Friday was an 'academic day' when, after doing the rounds of his post-operative patients, he could write and read, do paperwork, and be at home for his children.

Within months of his return to work in Sydney, journalists were chasing him again and he wasn't hard to catch. A talented, charismatic and talkative surgeon is a rare resource for the media and their audiences. In May 2000, the television program *Good Medicine* showed Charlie doing a sixteen-hour operation on a child with a large tumour who had been turned away by another doctor. His office immediately received phone calls from all over the country. Many were from Perth, Genevieve's home town, from parents of children whose brain tumours had been treated unsuccessfully by local neurosurgeons. In Charlie, they saw another chance.

Daniel Jordan, a fifteen-year-old schoolboy, had been diagnosed with tumours in his brain and spine when he was eleven. He lost control of his left arm and developed a limp in his left leg as the tumours grew. Eighteen months of chemotherapy followed by radiotherapy and surgery to remove some of the tumours saw no improvement. The Perth doctors told Daniel's parents that it was too dangerous to remove his fast-growing brain tumour, which had now become malignant, and that he had six months to live.

That was when the Jordans saw Charlie on television. After studying Daniel's scans, Charlie agreed to operate. He warned Daniel that he could die on the operating table or come out paralysed but, left untouched, the tumour would certainly kill him. In July 2000, Charlie performed three operations on the boy, totalling forty hours, and removed ninety-five per cent of the tumour along with the part of his brain that controlled movement on his left side. To Charlie's amazement, Daniel survived with no more disability than before the surgery. His tumour, it turned out, was not malignant but a rare, low-grade variety.

Daniel's father, Ray Jordan, was deputy editor of the *West Australian* newspaper. He wrote about their experience, and the paper ran news stories about Daniel and several other Perth patients who had turned to Charlie.

The parents of three-year-old Lily Glaskin had almost given up after her brain stem tumour returned despite two operations and chemotherapy. Charlie removed the tumour and promised to operate again if it reappeared. Another boy, twelve-year-old Daniel Monks, was permanently paralysed in the right arm and leg by a biopsy that damaged nerves and resulted in swelling and haemorrhage in the spinal cord. His parents were told the tumour was inoperable, but they had read about Daniel Jordan's success and took their son to Charlie Teo, who removed the tumour – a low-grade astrocytoma – with no further deficit and no recurrence.

Charlie didn't promise miracles – Lily Glaskin would later die from the return of her tumour – but Daniel Jordan and Daniel Monks went on to lead active lives.

In July 2001, the *West Australian* ran another series of stories, this time claiming that Perth doctors were refusing to refer patients to Charlie. 'Parents should be given all the information and have the chance to decide what options they take,' said Daniel Monks' mother, Annie Murtagh-Monks. 'They should be welcoming with open arms someone like Charlie Teo who has come from a major neurosurgical hospital in the United States but instead they think he's a cowboy and they won't go near him. It is in spite of the health system in WA that we have ended up with a positive outcome.'

Four Perth neurosurgeons, none of whom had been named in the articles, took such offence at the criticism that they lodged a complaint against Charlie with the Royal Australasian College of Surgeons. In their gratitude and anger, the parents of Charlie's patients had made comparisons that the four surgeons considered damaging to their reputations. Charlie had not personally criticised them, though one story had made it seem so, and the only grievance he ever aired publicly was against doctors who refused to refer patients to him. Nevertheless, the Perth group launched a campaign to have him deregistered.

When Aaron McMillan's life was placed in his hands in August 2001, Charlie was under siege. He sat in his pink-walled office and studied the brain scans. If Aaron died or was left seriously disabled by surgery, as Charlie was sure he would be, there were people who would use the case as evidence of his arrogance and fallibility. At forty-three, he could see his hard-built career blowing up. He worked well under pressure but not under that kind of pressure. He didn't want to be seen as rushing into an impossible mission, and he didn't want to be the one who ended Aaron's dreams. It would be much better for someone else to take the case.

He took the scans into Bernard Kwok's office and said, 'Bernie, would you mind taking over? Or can we do it together?'

'No,' replied the unflappable Hong Kong–born Kwok. He reasoned that this was a tough case for any neurosurgeon and a poor outcome wouldn't reflect badly on Charlie. He believed Charlie was the person most capable of succeeding.

Charlie was grateful but he still wanted help. Aaron's case was presented at grand rounds, the Monday afternoon session where the surgeons discussed their work with colleagues. Charlie was operating and couldn't attend, but Sami Harik, who was now professor and chairman of neurology in Little Rock, Arkansas, was visiting that week. He listened, examined the scans and said that, based on his knowledge of Charlie's work, if anyone could do the surgery, he could. The other neurosurgeons agreed that Charlie would not be to blame if such a tricky case went wrong. Certainly, no one else offered to take it over from him.

The truth was, however much they disapproved of Charlie's unorthodox behaviour, even his antagonists could not find fault with his skill, his courage and his results as a clinical neurosurgeon. Many of his colleagues thought he was the most outstanding brain tumour surgeon in the country. Some of them just couldn't bear to say so.

6

PRELUDE IN D

The story of Aaron McMillan and Charlie Teo has an eclectic soundtrack. Beethoven segues into Abba, Elvis collides with Chopin, Xenakis meets INXS. Although they had vastly different tastes they both needed music.

Whatever the coming days brought, Aaron didn't want to live without his piano. Back in the security of Ward 8, on a higher dose of dexamethasone and analgesics, he slept and his distress passed. Charlie came in on his morning rounds, disappointed that Aaron couldn't do without heavy medication and hospital care. Yet he was not to be treated as an invalid. Charlie said that for Aaron to stay stable – to stay alive – he had to be mentally active. The worst thing he could do was to curl up into a ball of self-pity. Charlie agreed with evidence that showed a positive attitude strengthened the immune system, lifted the spirits and helped people to survive.

There was still a week to go until Aaron's embolisation, booked for Wednesday 15 August. That time could either be wasted in fear or lived fully with his family and his friends, his music and his business, making sense of his life and reaching as far into the future as possible. Aaron asked if he could have his piano in the ward. His request went against hospital regulations, and normally the logistics would have made it impossible, but with so many rooms sitting empty, everyone agreed it was an inspired idea. The upright electric piano that Aaron kept in his apartment for practice was heavy but portable and could be used with headphones and volume control so as not to disturb other patients.

Ashley Eastwood gave her permission, provided Aaron did not move the piano into his shared room and that he used headphones 'at all times'. His father borrowed a van and wrestled the instrument up to the eighth floor, down the corridor and into a faded room that held nothing but a few limp metal fittings and the ghosts of patients past.

Now Aaron set himself a number of tasks. One was to learn Prelude in D by Sergei Rachmaninov, his favourite piece of music but one he had never bothered to master without a score. Listening to the simple two-note opening melody unfolding in typical sonata form and developing towards a huge, stately climax, Aaron felt he was watching the earth turn from outer space. Its grandeur fitted with his expansive way of thinking and his belief in a powerful force, greater than all of us. If he was going to learn one more piece before he died, it would be this one.

Prelude in D was the only piece of music he practised while in hospital, four pages over and over. It was the first time he had allowed himself the fun of endlessly repeating a single bar or phrase. He was usually under deadline for a performance or a recording but now he concentrated on his fingering and the dynamics of the sound.

Before long, he thought, 'Bugger it, I'm going to live. I'm going to play this.'

Day and night, he would take what felt like a long walk down to the 'spooky' end of the ward, the deserted rooms where he and his piano created a spot of vibrant energy. Although he was playing for himself at first, the headphones rule was never enforced and his tunes carried on the disinfected air to the patients and staff.

A study conducted at London's Chelsea and Westminster Hospital between 1999 and 2002 found the level of the stress hormone cortisol was forty-eight per cent lower in patients who had been exposed to soothing visual art or live music than in those who had not experienced either. Anxiety was thirty-two per cent lower and depression thirty-one per cent lower in patients after listening to music. A German doctor, Ralph Spintge, has in recent years assembled similar data on one hundred and fifty thousand surgical and pain patients. He found that if he played music during certain clinical procedures he could reduce the patients' subsequent drug dosages by half because the biochemistry of their blood was altered.

Formal music therapy grew out of the discovery during the two world wars that veterans' psychological and physiological health improved after hearing live music played in the hospital wards. However, the connection between health and the arts goes back at least to the ancient Greeks. Apollo, the god of music, poetry, healing and light, was the father of Asclepius, god of medicine. Even the most unscientific listener can sense the power of music to calm or stimulate the emotions and the body. As well as entering the brain, the sound resonates inside the body, keeps time with the heartbeat and stirs the most primitive emotions. 'Music,' writes Oliver Sacks in *Musicophilia*, 'uniquely among the arts, is both completely abstract and profoundly emotional'.

Aaron had always thought of his music as the most direct way to communicate. Without planning, he turned his ward into a recital hall.

After his dramatic return to hospital, he had a new room and a new roommate. Eighty-year-old emphysema patient Arnold Taylor had wound up in the neurosurgery ward because in winter there were never enough beds for the respiratory and old-age patients. Lying in his bed by the window, coughing and feeling ghastly, he looked up and saw a young bloke walk in with his mother and a few friends.

'He doesn't look too bad,' Arnold thought, envious of his youth. When he heard Aaron ask about getting hold of a CD player, he silently cursed, 'Good God, not bloody rock'n'roll.'

Whether he lived or died, Aaron was determined to complete his CD. When Yossi Gabbay visited, Aaron asked him to finish the editing if he didn't come back from surgery. He had an office set up on his bed. With a phone, a calendar and people running errands, he made plans for everything he would do when he left hospital and plans for everyone else if he didn't. He listened over and over to the music he had recorded. Behind the pink curtain, Arnold listened too – he had no choice – and was surprised at the pleasure it gave him. He was no classical music buff, but he floated on the tunes and felt soothed by the clear, warm voice of the piano.

'A bit of a piano player, are you?' Arnold asked when Aaron poked his head around the curtain.

Once he knew Aaron was a professional pianist, Arnold listened more carefully. He was confined to bed and couldn't shuffle along to hear Aaron play in what was becoming known as the piano room. But many others did. As more visitors came, Aaron often found it convenient to herd them out of his room and down the corridor for an impromptu concert. Once he started playing, nurses and patients drifted in and smiled at the pale, tousled figure bent over his keyboard.

Among his audience on Friday 10 August were Rosemary and Stuart Gentle, a couple who had taught at Glenaeon Rudolf Steiner School, where Aaron had been a pupil, and had watched him grow as a man and a musician. When Aaron asked what Rosemary would like to hear, she said, 'Play your favourite.' He gave them the Rachmaninov prelude.

It was difficult to imagine they might not hear him again, that his talent could be silenced. As the Gentles drove home, they talked about finding a way to record the story of his music and his courage so they would live on even if Aaron didn't.

On the outside, Aaron seemed remarkably like his usual self as he shared his music, cups of tea and conversation with his visitors. Inside, he had begun an intense self-examination. He had always tried to make sense of why things happened to him when they did, what an experience was trying to tell him. But what good could come from having a brain tumour? Already he had travelled from the panic of the first bewildering days to a more rational state. He did not pray, exactly, but conducted a very deliberate internal dialogue with a power that he thought of as God and also as his higher self. While not conventionally religious, he had a strong personal philosophy that had grown out of all the influences of his childhood and filtered through his own determined nature.

For Aaron this was the emotional climax of his illness, where his mind – not just his brain – found the necessary defences for the coming battle. It would be calm and stately, rather like the musical climax of the Rachmaninov piece before it falls from its pinnacle and changes key.

'I was definitely dealing with this individual presence – God, I suppose – praying, talking, trying to have some guidance,' he recalled later. 'It was like a test, a real examination. I felt very strongly that this force was telling me something quite hard to take but I knew I had to deal with it. It was saying, "Figure out what it is that you're here to do. Stop wasting your time. Stop using up the earth we've put you down on. Be focused and get your priorities sorted out or without doubt we will take you off." That was so much what I was being told: if I didn't resolve it, if I didn't come up with fire in my belly and a determination to get on with it and focus on the long-term path, then it was, "Sorry, Mr Young Employee, but you've been wasting your time and ours".

'Not once did I have personal thoughts that I want to grow up and have a family and have a life. There was this on-a-mission feeling. Everything else had to come second. I had to convince myself and [convince] this entity I was communicating with that this was what I was here for, that life was extremely precious and that I had to make the most of it, to contribute what I have, which is music. It wasn't a situation where before I had been out with girls and taking drugs – I was never like that. I felt I was trying but just not enough.'

Aaron was being hard on himself. For a 24-year-old he had an impressive curriculum vitae. But behind all the practice and performance and prizes, he had long been convinced there was a greater reason for the music that ran through him. Now was the time to define it.

7

PIANO MAN

No one recognised Aaron as an especially musical child, though he showed some early signs. There is a photograph of him sitting on an uncle's knee as a baby, plinking on the keys of a piano. His grandparents remember his songs filling their house. On his first aeroplane flight he sang all the way from Sydney to Griffith to hide his fear and a nun complimented him on his sweet voice, and at four he taped a collection of his favourite songs and stories, delivered with confidence, for his unknown father. Gail promised to send it to him and, if she had, it would surely have melted Brian's heart. But the tape stayed at Frank and Marjorie's house, as Gail was convinced that Brian would only have lost it. There's a story that Gail took piano lessons when Aaron was three or four and as he lay in bed listening to her make the same mistake in Bach's *Anna Magdalena* minuet night after night, he vowed to play the piece properly one day. Aaron couldn't remember that early determination and didn't give the piano any serious thought until he was past the age when most professionals are showy little performers.

He was born on 11 February 1977, the fruit of a short, passionate affair between Gail Robinson and Brian McMillan, who had met while living in a Buddhist household in Sydney's inner-west suburb of Glebe. They were looking for spiritual enlightenment and not planning to leave with a bundle of responsibility. Gail was a young schoolteacher, and Brian had dropped out of university after a motorbike accident and was drifting through odd jobs as a courier and welfare worker. They lived together until Gail's pregnancy crystallised Brian's feelings of inadequacy. He was not ready for fatherhood. Though he was present at Aaron's birth, Gail barely saw him afterwards and told him to go away, find himself and come back when he could be useful. He left for Thailand in search of nirvana when Aaron was fifteen months old, and didn't return for sixteen years.

Gail raised Aaron alone and went back to teaching when he was one. They lived in a series of rented homes; their security was with Gail's parents in the solid family house constructed by Frank's building company in the southern suburb of Penshurst. Aaron had love and attention from the three adults, with Frank filling the paternal gap. Marjorie, with her natural, selfless energy, was the person Aaron quickly came to see as his guiding light. As a single mother, Gail wanted everything for her son, but sometimes she seemed more like a slim, long-haired sister who was still growing up herself.

When Aaron was six she took him to New Zealand to pursue her growing interest in Steiner education. By then she had travelled mentally from her parents' devout Catholicism to Buddhism and anthroposophy, a spiritual science developed by the Austrian philosopher Rudolf Steiner, who described it as 'a path of knowledge leading the spiritual in the human being to the spiritual in the universe'. Aaron was enrolled in year one at the Steiner school where Gail studied. It was a time of bonding for mother and son, which ended with a drive around New Zealand in a Mini Minor, running perilously short of money, and surviving a storm and a shattered windscreen.

Life back in Sydney was marked by frequent house moves as Gail established her independence, balanced by the steadiness of Glenaeon, the Steiner school at Middle Cove, overlooking the harbour from its northern shore.

Steiner education emphasises imagination, independent learning, awareness of self and kindness to others, qualities Aaron would carry into his adult life. He was a sunny, playful boy, a quick student, a daring BMX bike rider and a skilled cubbyhouse builder in the bushland playground. He took the role of the hare in a school performance of Aesop's fable 'The Hare and the Tortoise'. He loved calculating numbers and constructing cities with his Lego blocks. His projects were always ambitious. When the class learned to knit a patchwork square, Aaron knitted on until he had a full-size jumper. The kindergarten still has a rug he wove while waiting for Gail to collect him after her classes. On one wall of his grandparents' garage he marked out a huge grid and in paints copied a picture of a fighter plane like the ones his grandfather flew in World War II.

Gail met Giles Puckett, a computer software designer, when Aaron was seven. Although surprised to hear there would be a stepfather and a baby, Aaron was also thrilled at the prospect of having a settled family and home in the bushy northern suburb of Forestville. He liked Giles, and was happy to see his mother content. He would love having a brother, Andrew, and later a sister, Amy. After school he hurried home to play with them, helped change nappies, read stories, baked birthday cakes and felt responsible for balancing the household, a bit like a second dad. When Amy was seven he worked until 3 am on Christmas Day to set up a new trampoline for her in the living room as a present from Santa Claus.

Like most primary school-age children, Aaron had learned to toot on the recorder. Steiner teaches that at the age of nine a child has the discipline needed to study a musical instrument seriously. Gail decided to introduce Aaron to the piano after consulting a musician who said he had good hands. His school friend, Nick Flint, who was already learning third-grade piano, often played at lunchtime and the music flowed down the corridor. Aaron watched him running through pieces by Muzio Clementi and Carl Czerny and wanted to produce the same kind of sound. Nick Flint turned his attention to playwriting and later joined the Sydney Theatre Company. Aaron showed some writing skill too and at sixteen the two boys won a New South Wales Children's Week award for a work about family, school and nature, called *All the World's a Play*, which they wrote, directed and produced.

Through the school, Gail organised lessons with a local teacher, Coral Paterson, and, with help from Giles and Frank, bought a piano for two thousand dollars. Aaron learned excellent technique from Paterson: she taught him to hold his hand over the keyboard as if cupping a tennis ball and, unlike many students, he never let his wrists sag. He could sight-read with ease, as though he had always spoken the language of music.

When he was ten he composed a piece of music to celebrate the birth of his brother, Andrew, and within three or four years had filled a pile of exercise books with fifty compositions, many so complex that he left them unfinished. He spent four months on an opera based on a book, *The King of Ireland's Son* by Padraic Colum, writing eighteen score pages based on just seven of the book's four hundred and sixty pages before he gave up.

Aaron quickly became the star pianist at Glenaeon, giving concerts and winning national prizes and scholarships. A few weeks before his eleventh birthday, his great-aunt heard him perform and afterwards wrote to Gail: 'Oh, what a god-given talent, in one so young. He is also a beautiful soul. This is no ordinary person. The gods have sent him for some special mission, and I do believe he knows this. You are a very lucky girl indeed, to be so chosen, but you will also have a tough time ahead . . .'

Aaron was eager to increase his musical skills and knowledge. When he bought his first CD, Bach's *French Suites* played presto by the idiosyncratic pianist Glenn Gould, it was to improve his own reading of the music. He was learning seventy pieces at once, with an A–Z chart on the wall to record his progress, and setting himself exercises: play all thirty-two Beethoven sonatas in one weekend; find the moment when the Classical period gave way to the Romantic.

School mates admired him both as an entertainer and a leader. As a teenager, he went on an Outward Bound camp, seven days in the wilderness which were meant to teach the teenage participants self-reliance and practical skills. But within days, the group was panicking and a boy was carried out with a broken leg. Aaron could see the need to take charge. With his map and compass, he plotted a way out of the bush. He cooked meals for everyone. The others took to asking, 'Aaron, what are we doing next?' At the end of the week, the adults saw Aaron come over the hill with a stream of kids behind him. He received a special commendation for his calm resourcefulness.

However, music engaged Aaron so completely that he paid dwindling attention to his school work and social life. His passion for music was matched only by his passion for basketball. As a tall, agile teenager, playing guard and forward, he was probably an even better sportsman than musician. At fourteen he was so keen on the game that the tip of every finger was continually cut and bleeding from bouncing the ball. The next year he captained his local team to a state premiership win and was named Most Valuable Player. When he started to think about playing for Australia at the 2000 Olympics he knew it was decision time: basketball or piano?

During a training session one day, Aaron ran and leaped to throw himself between another player and the ball. Coming down, he landed on the other boy's foot, lost his balance and crashed to the floor. There was an awful cracking sound. He was carried off to hospital in agony with a compound fracture – half a dozen breaks in one ankle.

For the next six weeks he was at home with his foot in plaster, poking at his itchy ankle with a knitting needle and missing the basketball trials. He was also headed for his eighth-grade piano exam. So he pushed his bed into the room where the piano stood and started practising; he would learn the left-hand part of a piece, then turn his whole body around on the bed and learn the right-hand part. Ten weeks after his fall he gingerly walked back onto the basketball court and knew that that phase of his life was over.

Many great artists have developed their talent after illness cut off other options and enforced bed rest gave them time to think creatively. Marcel Proust was a party boy until chronic asthma kept him indoors, sleeping by day and working at night on his vast literary masterpiece, *Remembrance of Things Past*. The painter Henri Matisse worked as a law clerk before an attack of appendicitis at twenty confined him to bed and his mother gave him a paint box to save him from boredom.

Aaron's epiphany was smaller but just as clarifying. From now on he would devote himself to music. Coral Paterson, his teacher, advised him to move slowly through the grades; she had plans to take him to study in Italy, but he became impatient.

He had already skipped every grade permissible and now he went for the eighth-grade exam with all his pieces perfectly memorised. When he arrived, ready to play, the examiner asked, 'Where are your music sheets?' He hadn't brought them because he had no need of them. But she was immovable: no music, no exam. Aaron ran out of the room, shocked and swearing. This setback increased his determination. Instead of taking another year to progress to ninth grade for his Associate Diploma in Music (AMus), he would do the exams for eighth grade, ninth grade and the final tenth grade, for the Licentiate Diploma (LMus), all within six months.

Wondering how to achieve his goal, Aaron made contact through a friend's father with the distinguished conductor and music educator Richard Gill. On Gill's recommendation he visited Neta Maughan, one of Australia's most respected piano teachers. She had studied with Alexander Sverjensky, who traced a line of teachers back to Rachmaninov and Liszt, and in turn taught young stars such as Michael Kieran Harvey, Simon Tedeschi and her own daughter, Tamara Anna Cislowska.

Her rambling old house in Sydney's inner west was an ear-opening new world for Aaron. As he walked up the over-grown path for the first time, Tamara was thundering out a Rachmaninov prelude on the piano. Maughan burst through the door with a plastic bag wrapped around her foot, fussing about the broken plumbing.

Eventually she sat down beside the piano and asked Aaron to show her the program he was learning for his eighth-grade exam. Her first suggestion was to drop a Debussy piece because some examiners disliked the composer. As they went on, Aaron felt he had found a teacher with an exciting depth of knowledge and experience. In the end, he dropped the Associate Diploma and practised sixteen hours a day to go straight for the Licentiate Diploma later in the year.

Maughan was impressed by Aaron's ambition, talent and potential. He was a skilful sight-reader and his fingers moved easily around the keyboard. By now, aged sixteen, he was almost two metres tall, with long hands and fingers. While most concert pianists can play a ninth chord with one hand – stretching from thumb to little finger across nine white keys – Aaron could play an eleventh. He contrasted himself with Elton John, who complained that his chubby hands could only reach an eighth, which was a hindrance to his piano technique (though clearly he overcame the problem). But then there was Rachmaninov, who had the rare ability to play a twelfth and composed some pieces that he alone could perform.

Exam day was 7 October 1993, his grandmother's birthday. Aaron went to the Sydney Conservatorium to play for Warren Thomson, chairman of the Sydney International Piano Competition, and two other examiners. At the piano that day he decided on the performance style he would continue to use: engage the listeners by giving everything possible in the first bar, the first page, the first piece; the rest will take care of itself.

He threw himself into his Bach piece and forgot his opening nerves, then began a Schubert sonata, wondering what he would do if they wanted to hear the third and fourth movements, which he hadn't had time to memorise. Thomson stopped him at the end of the second movement and said, 'That's great; that's enough.' He finished with a Chopin scherzo and breezed through the sight-reading and general knowledge questions. When he walked out into the sunshine, his family was waiting to celebrate with a picnic in the Botanic Gardens.

Aaron was stunned by his results: not only had he passed but he was the youngest pianist to earn the LMus with distinction that year. A photograph shows a lanky Aaron in his robes at the awards ceremony beside tiny twelve-year-old Simon Tedeschi, who was there to receive his AMus and would beat Aaron by gaining the LMus with distinction the following year.

Aaron's success raised him into the elite of Maughan's students and brought an array of opportunities. Thomson, his examiner, had noted that he played Schubert with tremendous originality and invited him to participate in the next Sydney International Piano Competition, in 1996. Before that he performed almost constantly in events around Australia. He and Cislowska won the Sydney Two Piano Competition together, and sneaked their first kiss, though her mother disapproved of any intimacy between her star pupils.

During that momentous year, Aaron met his father for the first time since his move to Thailand. Brian's mother had died; Gail had written saying her son needed a father; and finally Brian had decided it was time to return to reality. Aaron had kept a photograph of Brian dressed in his monk's saffron robes and often imagined he would fly to Thailand to find his dad, show him his birthmark and say, 'Look, it's me. I'm your son.'

Instead, Gail drove him to Bondi, where Brian was staying with his sister, Dene. Aaron thought he was a pleasant, gawky guy and impressed him by playing a flashy piece of Beethoven on Dene's piano. They discovered over the next few years that they both liked cricket, golf and movies. But from there father and son differed: while laidback Brian would move to a Buddhist monastery in the Southern Highlands, finding occasional work as a cook and handyman, Aaron was busy with a career that was going in a multitude of directions.

8

THE MECHANIC

Bent over, wielding his instruments, Charlie Teo could almost be mistaken for a motor mechanic. Drills, forceps, scissors, knives, screwdrivers lined up beside him; the inert body under his hands. Brain surgery is, at first glance, a manual skill, and there was a brief time after finishing school when Charlie did indeed work as an apprentice car mechanic. As a child, while his parents tried to interest him in playing the piano and other aesthetic pursuits, his hobbies had all centred around making things: Lego, Meccano sets, model aeroplanes. As an adult, he would renovate a house and rewire another.

Charlie was the son of immigrants from Singapore. Philip Teo, an obstetrician-gynaecologist, and Elizabeth, a nurse, met as students at King George V Hospital in Sydney. Though brought up in a Buddhist family, Dr Teo senior was a devout Anglophile and the couple completed their royal set by naming their children Charles and Anne. They lived in a modest fibro house at Picnic

Point in the city's far southern suburbs, where Charlie and his sister shared a tacked-on bedroom. Philip Teo's ambition was for his son to be a doctor and, at four years old, Charlie was sent to one of the city's elite private schools, Trinity Grammar.

Early one morning, little Charlie jumped into his parents' bed and pointed out the window. 'Daddy, Daddy, I want to do that.' Outside, the dunny man was going past, carrying the pan from the neighbours' unsewered toilet.

'I'm paying so much and that's what your son wants to be . . .' said the disappointed father.

Charlie's mother knew better: it was the dunny man's muscles her son admired. Charlie felt pressure from her, too, to be a doctor but she told him he could be a coolie if he liked, as long as he was no problem to her or to the government. His grandmother called him 'Prince Charles' and advised him to be a doctor rather than a lawyer, because he would never be able to sleep knowing he defended criminals.

Elizabeth Teo was raised as a Christian and took on her husband's Buddhism. She is a tiny woman with a huge will, a black-and-white view of right and wrong, and a tough approach to childrearing. Charlie was a good boy but so quiet she described him as 'a blob'. Instead of giving him pocket money, she sent him out to work in the holidays, doing a milk run and pumping petrol. She secretly paid the garage owner to employ him at first, insisting that he make Charlie clean the toilets and keep his wage low. Her aim was to teach him the tedium of menial jobs, so that he would work hard at school and become a professional. But the lesson almost backfired; he enjoyed learning how to operate a bowser, talking to customers and, later, picking up mechanical skills.

The adult Charlie adheres to no particular religion. He

describes himself as loosely Buddhist and credits his mother with teaching him the principles that guide him in life. Her lessons were simple but uncompromising. Treat other people as you would like them to treat you. Don't think you're above anyone else. You can always learn from others, so listen carefully. Communicate well with ordinary folk, because they're who will influence the sort of person you are and whether you succeed or not. Be acutely honest, even if it gets you into hot water. And the higher you fly, the further you will fall.

When Charlie was nine, his father went to study in England and had an affair with another woman, whom he would later marry. She was also called Elizabeth and their sons would be named Andrew and Edward. At home, there was a prolonged, acrimonious break-up. Charlie stood up for his mother and took some severe beatings from his father until he refused to see him. The two men reconciled when Charlie was in his forties, shortly before Philip's death. Charlie felt some sympathy for the old man at his funeral, where he heard for the first time that as a child in Singapore after the Japanese invasion, Philip had learned Japanese so that he could survive and make his way in the world.

Charlie missed having a father to show him how to hammer a nail and guide him into manhood. He looked everywhere for role models and authority figures. He admired some of the boys at school who were good sportsmen, but often they were disappointing off the field. He couldn't find what he needed in teachers or other boys' fathers. But he found it on television.

Dr Kildare, the infallible American surgeon played for years by the actor Richard Chamberlain, had a profound effect on Charlie. In one episode, Dr Kildare needed very steady hands to remove a tumour from a patient's head. Charlie went to his Lego set, built a model and practised reaching in to remove a piece of

Lego without touching the sides. From then on he set himself exercises to develop a firm hand in case he ever had to remove a tumour or disarm a bomb.

Bruce Lee, the kung fu star, appealed to his aggressively physical side. Charlie took up karate at nine and had his black belt before he turned eighteen. He liked the bodily discipline and mental concentration it gave him, as well as the muscles. But his greatest hero was John Wayne, the handsome, laconic cowboy who always coped when things went bad. As a boy, he admired Wayne's unshakable strength; as a man, he found it in himself.

At twenty-three and living with Genevieve in their first house at Balmain, he was frying chips in their kitchen one night when the pan of oil overheated and caught alight. The curtains blew up, and the fire lapped at the ceiling and turned everything brown. Charlie made the mistake of throwing water on the oil, which made the flames leap higher, and then put a tea towel over it and that caught fire too. He was still clear-headed enough to stand back and ask himself, 'What would John Wayne do now?' He decided John Wayne would go outside and get some sand from the garden to dowse the fire. That was the first time his hero saved him.

After his father left, Charlie was sent as a boarder to Scots College in distant Bellevue Hill, a Presbyterian private boys' school overlooking Sydney Harbour, where he would be well educated, wear a straw boater and play the bagpipes in the cadet band. He was in the first schoolboy contingent invited to the Royal Military Tattoo in Edinburgh, and as a surgeon he would dress up in his kilt to play in the children's ward, at his sister's wedding, and in the Scots old boys' band for the Anzac Day march. As a company sergeant major in the band, he was taken aside by a teacher and advised that, while his high standards were admirable, he was expecting too much of the other students. He knew it was a character flaw, but ever afterwards he would demand excellence from his family, colleagues and staff.

Among his peers at school, he felt like a daggy misfit. He was one of only two or three Asian boys in his year, a clever student, and an amusing and sometimes outrageous second speaker on the debating team. He played Charley in a school production of the English farce *Charley's Aunt*. He was sinewy and athletic but preferred karate to football. He had no fashion sense, dressing in high-waisted jeans, and his favourite singer was the caftan-wearing Indian-Australian Kamahl until two girlfriends took him in hand. He wasn't into girls in the sniggering way of teenage boys and when the crowd headed off to the pub, Charlie would more likely go with a friend to a Chinese restaurant for dinner. Inevitably, there were rumours that he was gay. The simple truth was that he never drank alcohol and he *loved* to eat.

His classmate Trevor Danos often invited him home at weekends and the family noted his bottomless pit of a stomach. They always sent him back to school with tins of food. Years later, Trevor watched Charlie complain about the small portions at an Italian restaurant and rise to the owner's challenge: if he could finish an enormous bowl of pasta, his meal was free. Even now, he devours his mother's hot Singaporean curries, loves cooking for friends at home, and it is not unusual, after a long day's surgery or after a full meal, for him to gather a bunch of colleagues and head to Chinatown for pork buns.

Charlie's appetite for life, his warmth, openness and lack of snobbery have always endeared him to a wide range of people.

The night in January 1976 when the university entrance results were published, a group of his schoolfriends drove him to the old *Sydney Morning Herald* building at Broadway and saw him cartwheel with joy at finding his name on the noticeboard among the few accepted for medicine at the University of New South Wales. He was proud to have succeeded, and to have fulfilled his mother's expectations, yet he still wasn't convinced that he wanted to be a doctor.

Since his early ambition to empty dunnies, Charlie had also considered becoming a full-time karate instructor, a politician or a lawyer. While some of his friends took off on holiday before university, he still needed to earn money. He started as a groundsman at Scots College, but that quickly bored him, so he moved on to his job as a car mechanic. He enjoyed the manual work and the achievement of fixing engines so much that he thought about foregoing medicine. However, he knew that underneath a car there would be little interaction with other people. He would miss that. And then one day a customer came in and asked him a question that he couldn't hear over the noise in the workshop. Thinking he couldn't understand because he was Chinese, she repeated her question, carefully enunciating the words as if she were talking to an idiot. That tinge of racism was a warning. Charlie was offended and realised that, even though he believed in treating everyone equally, there were people who would treat him according to his status. He wanted respect. Maybe his parents had been right all along.

At university, Charlie's personal style began to emerge. He moved into Basser College and then into a flat with his girl-friend, Maree, who was studying physiotherapy. He began riding a motorbike, and earned his pocket money as a karate instructor and as a barman-cum-toilet cleaner and bouncer at the

Centrepoint Tavern in the city. He sang in a band called the Old 57s. The daggy teenager developed an edge.

Once in medicine, he was drawn to the practical, manual skills of surgery. It was another way of fixing things. Because he liked children, he decided on paediatric surgery, but fooled around until he did six months in paediatric neurosurgery as part of the training rotation, and discovered his true calling. He had found the most physically, mentally and emotionally taxing specialty and also the newest. Neurosurgery was less than a century old and so little was known about the brain and its treatment that he believed he could still be a pioneer.

'The thing I love most about neurosurgery is it's a thinking man's specialty,' he once told me. 'So many times people think of surgeons as hackers: if in doubt cut it out; shoot from the hip; don't think too much. It's true: the surgeon's mentality is very much the jock from high school – the orthopaedic surgeon, good-looking guy, always been a good sportsman so he becomes a surgeon. It's physical and you don't need as many brains to do surgery as you do to do physician's training.

'That surgeon's mentality didn't appeal to me so I wanted to pick something where I could use my brains plus my hands. Neurosurgery was perfect. Not only is the actual surgery important but it's the planning, thinking about the case, the approach, all the different permutations and complications that can happen. You've really got to think hard, like [in] a chess game.

'Even to make an incision in the scalp is a bit more complicated because you've got to think about the cosmetics of it. If you make an incision in the wrong place, you cut off all the blood supply to the rest of the scalp. When you open up to get to the hip, you're just cutting through muscle so you can't really do much damage and it takes you about five minutes. Even when you're operating on the liver, you're just cutting through the anterior abdominal wall and it's skin and muscle and you don't have to think about it much and it takes about ten minutes. But to get to the head you've got to drill the bone off. Just that can kill the patient if you hit a major vein or penetrate the covering of the brain.

'Then, of course, when you get inside, the surgery is completely different too. Every blood vessel in the brain acts as an end artery. Once it's damaged, it's damaged usually for good, and you can't rectify that. You make a mistake and the patient dies or the patient's paralysed, or you make them a vegetable. So, the dictum in neurosurgery is that it's unforgiving. You can't make a mistake.'

9

DREAMS

To the dismay of his mother and schoolteachers and even his piano teacher, Aaron decided at seventeen that he didn't want to go to university and didn't need the Higher School Certificate. Music was everything. As he put it, 'I was in this new world, me and the piano, and music felt like an ocean compared to the teacup of school.' While he had maintained top grades in the early years of high school, now he was slipping. A teacher complained that it was hard to give him instructions because he was always composing under the desk. In year ten he scored twenty-eight per cent in chemistry. He left before the end of year eleven with a report that said, 'It seems as though Aaron's desire to continue his music has finally overtaken his desire to stay at school. We encourage his future.'

Aaron had no regrets. He focused on his study with Neta Maughan and for two months, to earn money, he taught thirty pupils of his own. Freed from school, family and other responsibilities, his entrepreneurial drive started to find outlets. For two years after leaving school at seventeen, he moved into the home of Julia Fluhrer, a music lover whose daughters, Johanna and Jen, were Glenaeon students. She had fallen in love with her 'little son' when she saw him playing the school's grand piano at twelve with a busker's bowl of coins collected from his listeners. As a schoolboy he went with her family on his first skiing holiday, broke her husband's ski poles getting off the chairlift and, stuck at the top, skied backwards down the mountain. It was clear Aaron couldn't be stopped and she admired his determination. Fluhrer presented him in piano recitals at her Wahroonga house in Sydney's north and in Adelaide, gave him the proceeds to save for a piano, bought him concert clothes and tried to teach him a deep stage bow. He would never give more than a dip of the head. While he was a charming, loyal and generous boy, she could see he craved fame and riches. His unconventional approach would take him on a meandering and sometimes manic journey for the next few years.

At the Sydney Town Hall in 1995, when his peers were preparing for the Higher School Certificate, Aaron brought together twenty Australian composers, including the veterans Miriam Hyde and Dulcie Holland, and the younger Mike Nock, Mark Isaacs and Elena Kats-Chernin, to perform their work. Having hired the hall and invited the participants, Aaron sat proudly in the audience; the concert was later broadcast on ABC Classic FM. For him, it was a landmark event that highlighted how few opportunities existed for Australian composers and musicians.

A younger cousin had been born with cystic fibrosis and as her health began to deteriorate that year, Aaron visited her in hospital every day for two weeks, playing tapes of Chopin nocturnes to distract her from her pain. After Susannah died, he recorded the two most beautiful pieces of music he knew – Liszt's B Minor Sonata and Schumann's *Fantasy in C* – for his first CD, dedicating it to his cousin and donating the proceeds to the Cystic Fibrosis Foundation.

A week after making the recording, he left for Europe with Sebastian Adams, a schoolfriend who would film his performances and moments between them. One film clip shows Aaron and a young German acquaintance cooking a messy breakfast of sausages, rice and 'screwed eggs'. In another, Aaron sits over a blank sheet of paper contemplating his future compositions and the sprawling creative process in which 'notes on a page' were only the final step.

Even as a child, Aaron had felt constrained by the twelve-semitone scale developed by J.S. Bach and used in all European music. It was as limiting as seeing only the twelve colours in the rainbow when, in fact, there are infinite colour variations. His creative ambition was to change the sound of music by developing new scales and a digital piano that could play them. In Germany, Aaron met the Romanian composer Horatio Radulescu, who was at the forefront of experimental work already being done to retune the scales. He and Aaron found that they both liked to work through the night, and Radulescu told how a friend had once kept him going with injections of vitamin C when he had to finish a concerto for the Frankfurt Symphony Orchestra.

At Beethoven's house in Vienna, Aaron was the only visitor in a room that was set up as if the composer still lived there. 'Would you like to play the instrument?' asked the woman in charge. Aaron sat down at Beethoven's piano and reverently played a movement of the *Moonlight Sonata*. He gave recitals in Vienna, Paris and Rome, and drove around Italy with another young traveller, visiting the catacombs and sneaking through secret corridors into a crowded midnight mass with Pope John Paul II at St Peter's Basilica. The climax of his trip was a month in Israel and a concert on Mount Carmel in Haifa, where his program included a sonata by Radulescu.

At home in 1996, encouraged by his encounter with the Romanian composer, he turned his energies back to writing his own music. Through Glenaeon and Gail, he had met David Wansbrough, a university lecturer, artist, poet and non-denominational clergyman with a passion for Russia. They shared an esoteric view of life's meaning with its foundation in anthroposophy, and Aaron suggested he might compose an orchestral piece based on David's poems. David was impressed by the boy's natural musicality and knowledge, and the way he radiated youth, but he doubted that the composition would eventuate. How could someone so young conjure music to lines such as 'I was the corpse that rolled in the sea's wash . . .'? Privately David wondered, 'What does he know? Has he met bitter disappointment, deep suffering, ennui?'

Over the next few months, Aaron wrote a thirty-minute symphonic poem, *For an Age Surf Tumbled*, for an eighty-piece orchestra and piano. He then assembled eighty musicians and a conductor to perform the work at the Willoughby Civic Centre in Sydney's north. His mother put in money, and served supper to the audience of three hundred. David Wansbrough sat mesmerised, his eyes closed, hearing the musical onomatopoeia of crying gulls and the rhythm of the sea. *The Sydney Morning Herald*'s veteran critic Fred Blanks wrote, 'If there is a prize for the year's most innovative concert, this one is in the running.'

Throughout 1997, Aaron performed furiously and made his first trip to South Africa. He had wanted to go since he was a small boy and told his grandparents about a vivid dream in which he was performing with African musicians in front of a huge festival crowd controlled by riot police. Over the years, he developed a real ambition to absorb the African musical cultures and work with African musicians to preserve their traditions. On the judging panel of the 1996 Sydney International Piano Competition, in which Aaron competed, was the chairman of the University of South Africa Music Foundation. Aaron was booked to travel to Spain the following year to play the *Iberia* piano suite by the Spanish composer Isaac Albeniz, and he decided to go via Pretoria. But he was dismayed at the apparent lack of contemporary African music. Even at the International Library of African Music, in Grahamstown, he found only a catalogue of recordings and instruments hung on the walls like museum exhibits.

Back home, on 3 July 1997 he hired the Sydney Town Hall to give a concert of piano improvisations based on more of the poems in David Wansbrough's collection *Dreams, Delights, Fears and Fragments*, and the following year released a CD of the concert with the actor Tom Burlinson reading Wansbrough's words. His networking and publicity skills were growing, and a thousand people filled the hall that night. Through David, Aaron met Lorenzo Montesini, a Qantas flight steward who was born in Alexandria and had a string of European titles. Lorenzo was chairman of the Australian Friends of the Library of Alexandria, supporting a new cultural centre on the site of the Egyptian institution that was destroyed some sixteen hundred years ago. He commissioned Aaron to write an anthem for the centre's planned opening and cultural collection. Aaron wrote *The Beacon*, based on *For an Age Surf Tumbled*, after visiting the waterfront city and the hole in the ground that would become the library. His main purpose in returning to Africa was to perform and to hear live African music at the Grahamstown Music Festival. This time he took his ten-year-old brother, Andrew, and between musical engagements they shared innumerable boys'-own adventures. A bullet brushed Aaron's arm as they dodged gunfire in Johannesburg. They hid in their car from a gang of baboons at a game park in Nairobi. Aaron bribed a guard to let him and Andrew climb one of the pyramids at night and they watched the sunrise from the top.

The return to Australia from this trip was less triumphant. Aaron's father had drifted back into the family's life, staying at the house in Forestville and spending time alone with Gail. Living at home again, Aaron saw Brian's presence as a threat to his secure family; he was angry with his mother and threw a punch at his father. His parents discovered strong remnants of the attraction that had brought them together twenty years earlier, and Gail and Giles separated. But Brian soon realised he still wasn't suited to domestic life and went back to the monastery at Bundanoon. Distressed and full of self-recrimination, in 2000 Gail packed her car and took Andrew and Amy with her to start a new life and teaching job in Brisbane. After a painful period for everyone, Giles moved to Brisbane and the family was reunited. Aaron was fiercely protective of his brother and sister, but when the turmoil subsided and his mother and siblings moved north, he chose to stay in Sydney, retreating to the womb of his grandparents' house before finding his own city apartment.

He hadn't acclimatised to normality after his African travels. He was tired and restless, finding performances difficult. He needed to step back, reflect on life so far and think about the next phase. He wondered later if the tumour had already started to intrude. Perhaps he was simply exhausted by the intensity of work he'd undertaken since he'd left school. While many of his old school friends were easing themselves into adulthood at university, Aaron was constructing a career out of his own talent, confidence and energy. Then there was the family drama, which had hurt everybody and left Aaron feeling resentful and alienated from his parents. Despite all his friendships, he hadn't found a serious girlfriend. After the tentative sexual moves of youth he didn't know how to meet girls or take the initiative. Sometimes he blamed his old school, where he had gone right through the years with a small group of girls who were like sisters. Any girls he liked now were either unavailable or uninterested; others he met left him unstirred. He was surprised that a concert pianist wasn't a magnet for women. A few times he went with friends to nightclubs or bars but nothing happened. However, he wasn't lonely, nor was he driven by sex. Perhaps women sensed that his mind was elsewhere.

As weary as he was over the next few years, he performed the *Iberia* piano suite around Australia, and gave a concert at the State Theatre in Sydney and then another ambitious performance at the City Recital Hall to celebrate the three-hundredth anniversary of the piano. Six hundred people attended that concert, and yet he and his supporters lost their money. Making a profit from classical music was hard but Aaron was undeterred. His ideas raced ahead of his ability to fulfil them. He set up a production and promotion company, Wayfarer, which he saw as a future vehicle for helping other musicians' career development. He registered the Australian Symphony Orchestra as a business name and planned to commission new works from Australian composers for international performance. After visiting Africa and Israel, he had decided that his vision fitted with the work of the United Nations. He contacted the United

Nations Association of Australia, whose members invited Aaron to be a local convenor for UNESCO and to perform at meetings. It was a first small step into world affairs.

He also allowed himself the new distraction of cricket. He had always felt the lack of a mentor, someone older who had achieved what Aaron was trying to do, who would push him to reach the highest standard and guide him in his career. Through his old school, he met some eleven-year-old boys who needed a cricket coach and, although Aaron hadn't played much cricket, he was a nifty bowler and a methodical strategist. He liked the idea of being the wise one who could help other people make the right moves.

Over three seasons, he turned a bunch of bumblers into a Manly district team that lost their final by just one run. Four of the eleven went on to the New South Wales under-fourteen squad. One of them was Jake Farriss, son of Tim Farriss, guitarist with the rock band INXS. Tim came closest to being a musical mentor. Even though their work was entirely different – Tim was an international rock star and didn't read music – he inspired Aaron with rock'n'roll's spontaneous energy, and the confidence with which the band recorded through the night in the studio, played in front of a Wembley Stadium crowd and brought out hit after hit the way some people went to the office.

One day at a cricket match, Aaron heard Tim talking to Jake about the boy's career plans. 'It's just a matter of getting on with whatever you want to do,' Tim said. 'People think it's hard. It's not too hard.'

To Aaron, searching for the secret of success, those simple words were a revelation. He could see that people often limited themselves by believing some goals were unreachable. He wanted to aim for the top and he was convinced that the magic qualities

needed to reach it were not talent or luck, but rather determination and effort.

As the new millennium began, Aaron was ready to refocus on
his life and his music. Hoping to sort out his finances and build
his audience, he planned his first truly commercial CD, to be
called *Time Within*. He asked everyone close to him to choose a
favourite piece of music for the collection, and began to practise
and record at the ABC. He could not anticipate the disruption
that was about to shatter his plans.

His star protégé was Elliot Bullock, a Mosman schoolboy who
was showing the passion for cricket that Aaron had for music.
When Elliot was thirteen, they planned how he would bat for
Australia by the time he was twenty-one. Elliott appreciated
Aaron's patient, organised style and in 2001, at the age of fifteen,
he was on schedule, playing fifth grade, and occasionally fourth,
for Manly.

At one of their training sessions at the Sydney Cricket Ground
that year, Elliot found his coach collapsed on the ground. He
didn't worry too much. It just seemed like a spot of dizziness
until, a few weeks later, Aaron phoned him from Prince of Wales
Hospital.

10

TWENTY-SIX HOURS

Good hands for a surgeon, as for a pianist, are strong and steady, light and agile, able to channel complex thought into unhesitating action. Peter Isert, an anaesthetist who has worked closely with Charlie Teo, sees Charlie's dexterity as a mixture of coordination, knowledge of anatomy, and something more: 'It's like his brains are in his fingers.'

Human fingers are such precise tools that the largest part of the motor cortex running across the top of the brain is devoted to controlling their movement. Neuroscience has not decided whether surgeons and pianists are more developed in that area than footballers or dancers. Charlie works at being physically fit and mentally disciplined, so he can stand and concentrate and pick away at a tumour for as long as it takes. His legs ache, his shoulders lock, but like an athlete he pushes through and ignores the pain until he crosses the finishing line.

Training, experience, a strong team and the best instruments all contribute to being an outstanding neurosurgeon. You have to be able to make a diagnosis and recognise the indications for or against surgery. But most important of all, in Charlie's view, is your mental attitude. If you care about a patient as a person rather than just a disease, he argues, you will not do anything recklessly harmful. And you will treat the person in both body and spirit.

Many times he has said, in slightly different ways, 'I have realised the power of the mind is incredibly important to your general wellbeing and the ability of the human body to fight disease. I don't know why doctors find this so hard to accept but they do. I think a lot of patients have done well not because I've operated on them, but because I've offered them hope and I've given them something to be positive about. It can't just be the surgery because anybody can do the surgery I do. They all leave in a very positive frame of mind: "We're going to beat this." I encourage that and I nurture it and I think it's instrumental. I think I have gained more understanding of the mind and the power of the mind not through looking at the brain, but through the dealings with my patients.'

Charlie's holistic philosophy is simple, logical and refreshing, but many doctors still find it unprofessional. He encourages his patients to exercise, follow a healthy diet, meditate, remain positive and, if they have religious beliefs, to pray. He also recommends surgery, sometimes repeatedly over many years, on tumours that others have declared inoperable or the operation pointless because the patient was going to die anyway.

Critics in the profession say Charlie gives false hope to hopeless cases with his pep talks and rush to operate. He argues that those surgeons often abandon patients when it is possible to save some and give many others more time, comfort and support. He makes it clear that a malignant tumour will ultimately prove fatal but that is no reason not to fight.

'While there's quality of life, there's hope,' he says. 'If people aren't willing to die, I will certainly not condemn them to a death sentence. People I've operated on that really should have died within six months, a lot of them are still alive and a lot survived two, three, four years. If you can give someone six months extra . . . who knows? The cure might be right around the corner.

'You tell people that their tumour could come back and if they want to absorb it, fine, but try not to focus on that. Focus on the fact that some people live and some people live a long time and why don't you just pretend you're that person? If you're going to be one of the people who lives four years instead of six months, wouldn't it be terrible to live those four years thinking, "Shit, I'm going to die next week," and four years comes up and you've wasted the time dying rather than living?'

Charlie talks at length with new patients, explaining their options, the possible outcomes, the pros and cons. Not everyone likes his exuberant, gung-ho approach. Some never return. Occasionally a patient complains that he didn't alert them to side effects, or that he could see only a surgical solution. A mother who took her child elsewhere says Charlie's diagnosis and surgery would have harmed her child. A former model who can no longer wear high heels claims Charlie did not warn her that surgery would leave her lame in one leg. Like all doctors, he can make mistakes. Although he is reluctant to say so, because doctors are always vulnerable, as I write this he has never been sued by a patient. Still, Charlie knows he's not for everyone; it's a matter of personality as well as medicine.

Most who take up his offer of radical surgery are grateful for the reprieve and rarely regret the decision. They do not accuse him of lying if the cancer recurs. To many, he is a hero. As one man put it, there is no such thing as false hope, only hope. Another who lived less than four months after surgery used the time to marry and have a honeymoon. He named his dog after Charlie. Two weeks before he died, he rang and said, 'Charlie, I'll see you in heaven. I just had a great sixteen weeks and I thank you for it.'

When he faces these patients, Charlie thinks back to a close friend who died of cancer as a young woman. Well-meaning visitors went to see her in hospital with promises to look after her children and other parts of her life when she was gone. She hated their kindness.

'Charlie,' she told him, 'the worst thing about dying is when you haven't given up but everyone else around you has. I want to keep fighting but it's a terribly lonely feeling.'

For a surgeon it is about persistence, in and out of the operating theatre. Charlie had learned that lesson as a medical student when he was doing a cardiothoracic term at St Vincent's Hospital in Sydney. A surgeon called Mark Shanahan headed the team that was replacing a patient's heart valve. The heart was diseased and flaccid, and every time Shanahan put a stitch into it the tissue would tear further. Charlie thought the patient was sure to die. But Shanahan wouldn't give up. Eventually, after hours of slippery attempts, he found enough solid flesh to make the stitches hold and the patient survived.

'How did you do that?' asked Charlie.

'Charlie, what makes a great surgeon rather than a good surgeon is perseverance.'

An ordinary brain tumour could be removed in two or three hours but Charlie took on the most difficult operations, which often lasted four or six hours or more. Then there were the marathons. His longest operation so far took twenty-six hours.

When he was working at the Children's Medical Center in Dallas, Texas, a fifteen-year-old girl arrived with an arterio-venous malformation, a large tumour completely made up of blood vessels. Charlie describes such tumours as 'very treacherous and they bleed like stink'. This one affected both the top and rear sections of the brain and was wrapped around the brain stem. Looking at it, Charlie thought there was no way he could remove it. But that didn't deter him.

For sixteen hours he worked with the precision of a jeweller. He had to burn each blood vessel with his bipolar forceps before cutting it so that he didn't provoke uncontrollable bleeding. There were thousands of tiny vessels. By midnight he was exhausted. His concentration wasn't waning but he hadn't drunk or eaten or urinated since early that morning. So when a more senior surgeon came into the theatre and suggested he take a break, he uncurled and left the patient in the other man's hands.

Urinating was painful after all those hours without fluids. Charlie had left a jug of lemon cordial and a chocolate ice-cream in the staff refrigerator for a quick energy boost. Now he was craving them. He gulped down the cordial and was about to bite into the ice-cream when a colleague ran in to call him back to the theatre. In the fifteen minutes he had been gone, the other surgeon had got into strife. The girl's brain had swollen and was bleeding profusely.

Charlie didn't blame his colleague. It was difficult to take over mid-operation – like a game of concentration where the cards are scattered all over the ground and you've memorised them, then you expect another player, who doesn't know what's under the cards, to take your place and win the game. Charlie moved in again, staunched the bleeding and continued the meticulous surgery for another ten hours. The girl woke up with a blind spot in her vision that was no worse than before the operation and recovered with no other ill effects.

As for Charlie, he felt great. After a session like that, which finished at ten o'clock the following morning, he just had time to go home for a shower before starting another day's work. He had the strange, jet-lagged feeling of having skipped a day. His only regret was that a friend of his wife had brought over homemade gumbo, the spicy southern stew, and they'd eaten every mouthful while he operated on an empty stomach. A decade later, he still moaned about missing the gumbo.

Even when everything seemed to go well, Charlie knew he didn't have total control. If ever he started to forget that, he reminded himself of a patient he encountered in 2000, soon after his return to Sydney. Jade was an eleven-year-old girl from northern New South Wales, who arrived at Prince of Wales with her grandparents after suddenly becoming ill. Her parents were overseas and by the time they flew into Sydney, Charlie had removed a brain tumour. She woke up smiling and Charlie was pleased with his work. Rather than send her straight home, he kept her and the family in Sydney for observation. But by the first evening, Jade had a headache and a bump under the wound on her head. Charlie thought there might be some internal swelling but nothing showed up on a scan. Then, without warning, Jade went rigid, began shaking and lost consciousness.

Seizures due to brain swelling are common after surgery and are not necessarily serious, but, although she recovered from the attack, Charlie admitted her to intensive care in case she suffered any more. She did have another seizure, and this time she didn't wake up. A ventilator didn't revive her. Charlie rushed in but the happy child he had seen half an hour earlier was limp, with fixed, dilated pupils. He had to walk out and tell her unsuspecting parents.

Charlie started bawling. For the first time in his career, he couldn't control his tears in front of a patient's family. Jade's parents were crying too but he couldn't comfort them. He couldn't talk. He stood in a corner and the pain engulfed him. He always felt the loss of a patient but Jade's death was unexpected and inexplicable. She reminded him of his eldest daughter, and she had worn her Chinese pyjamas in hospital just for Charlie.

He didn't go to the funeral, as he sometimes did. Jade's mother wrote a letter saying they appreciated his efforts; they didn't hold him responsible, but she would never recover from losing her daughter. Charlie tried to rationalise that Jade's type of tumour would probably have recurred in five or six years and she had been saved from a slow death. But he knew that wouldn't help her mother and it didn't help him.

Every month, doctors report bad results to their colleagues at a morbidity and mortality meeting, known in the profession as M&M. Charlie told Jade's story, explained that he had admitted and scanned her at the first doubt, and showed her X-rays so that other neurosurgeons could see there was no swelling or fluid. He had done everything by the book and he still had no idea what went wrong. The other doctors didn't blame him for her death, but she had been alive before he operated, so he blamed himself.

Jade's photograph stayed on the noticeboard in the children's ward for years. Charlie told her story wherever he travelled to teach his minimally invasive techniques. After presenting his excellent results, he flashed up the picture of Jade and added, 'Just remember, you can get bad results as well.'

In his office, Charlie has a sign that another neurosurgeon gave him: *In neurosurgery you're never on top of the world for more than ten minutes*. He hadn't understood the message at first, but after Jade's death he did. When you're operating on a human brain, things can go wrong as quickly as they can go right. You can never pat yourself on the back.

But Charlie believed too strongly in his mission to stay down. Patients streamed in from around Australia and the world, often referred by American doctors. He travelled to the United States six times a year to teach neuroendoscopy and, even when his students became qualified to teach, Charlie was surprised to find that they kept asking him back.

Every year since 1995, he had travelled with another doctor and a nurse to Lima, the capital of Peru, to operate pro bono at the only children's hospital in the country, and run a course in paediatric neurosurgery for local doctors. On the first day of each trip, he saw up to forty patients who needed treatment and, in a tough process of triage, chose about eight he could operate on over the next two days. He removed tumours and a pencil that had penetrated a child's brain through his eye. He treated children with hydrocephalus whose heads had become so distended with fluid they couldn't walk and had to be carried around in wheelbarrows. When the work was done he trekked with his colleagues and, on different trips, with his daughters Nicola and Alex, visited the ancient Inca ruins of Machu Picchu. Up there in the clouds, he felt closer to God.

11

A REASON TO LIVE

In the sunny stillness of an early morning in August 2001, before the clatter of hospital life began, Aaron lay in bed trying to visualise his future. He could see himself as a concert pianist or as the manager of a music company or as a composer. Unconsciously, he was preparing for a future when his body might not be fit for playing the piano or even running a business. But as he thought about the solitary art of composing, a rush of warmth passed through him. It was as if someone had said, 'Yes, that's right. Please focus on that because that's what you're here to do.'

He kept affirming that sense of purpose as if he were building muscles. He had a reason to live. It was the beginning of an answer to his metaphysical questions and now he could hand himself over to fate with a smile. Those around him noticed that he was no longer the anxious young man who had arrived at Emergency less than two weeks before.

Aaron's private concert in the ward jolted Rosemary and Stuart Gentle. Through their daughter, they contacted Ben Cheshire, a producer on *Australian Story*, the ABC television program that profiles ordinary individuals who have had remarkable lives. According to Ben, Aaron's story had the perfect formula: 'amazing pianist, wonderful guy, big tumour, not a very good prognosis, let's tell his story before it's too late'. He put to Aaron the idea of having a camera follow him through his operation. He found the young man surprisingly easygoing, even when Ben raised the awkward possibility that they might have to film his death.

'Yes, let's do it. Let's show them,' Aaron said.

An audience always energised Aaron and, if he could remain strong in front of the cameras, perhaps he could inspire others. If he lived, it was unbeatable publicity; for now, it was a welcome diversion. Each day he lived in front of the crew and the program's future audience. Perhaps he performed for them, putting on a little bravado, becoming an actor in his own drama.

When the cameras left, Arnold Taylor in the neighbouring bed saw Aaron at his most vulnerable, but never frightened or angry. He'd been shocked to learn about the gravity of his illness. This handsome boy, who played such beautiful music, couldn't possibly die. 'An old devil like me, I've had a good life,' he thought. 'But what's a young bloke like him being punished for?' They swapped life stories, chatted about cricket and, once or twice, when Aaron seemed despondent, Arnold cheered him up.

Arnold was a hospital veteran but he had never seen a room so crowded with flowers, balloons and cards. Then there was the procession of visitors, day and night. Aaron counted two hundred and forty in the two weeks leading up to his operation.

A few felt as if they were queuing at the bank and gave up. The nurses despaired of sticking to the permitted three at a time.

Aaron was putting his affairs in order, even though he didn't intend to die. Elliot Bullock and his cricket career represented the future and if Aaron couldn't guide him, he wanted to make sure someone else would. He asked Gavin Robertson, a former Australian Test cricketer he had met through Tim Farriss, to visit. It was a day when the cricket boys were playing Monopoly on a new board Aaron had bought for Elliot. The atmosphere was more like that of a picnic than a hospital room. When Gavin arrived, Aaron picked up the red apple from his dinner tray and handed it to him.

'That's what I've got in my head.'

He outlined his plan: 'Elliot wants to captain Australia one day. I'm feeling good but I've had to do a will and prepare for "what if" . . . What I've been for Elliot is a friend who loves cricket, someone who believes in you and is there if you need it.' Elliot, at the foot of the bed, listened with flushed cheeks as Aaron asked Gavin to take on the role.

Gavin promised he would. 'But I refuse to accept you won't be there.'

Arnold Taylor, listening in the next bed, thought, 'Here's a bloke looking at the pearly gates and he's worried about a little boy's career. Is he human?'

Spiritual support came to Aaron from a multitude of directions. His parents and grandparents meditated and prayed for him in their different ways. In Aaron's words, 'My grandparents are Catholic, my mother is sort of Catholic and I'm sort of sort of Catholic.' As a child he'd gone to mass, where he thought there was too much talk, and to Gail's Buddhist meetings, where he listened to the chanted 'om' and tried to work out what note it was. His real belief hung on his keyring: *Where words fail music speaks*. But he remained receptive to other people's faiths and the strength they offered him.

He often talked to another of Charlie's patients, a Yugoslav woman who walked the corridors with a breathing tube down her throat after surgery for a glomus jugulare tumour. Though she had lost some thirteen litres of blood, she was cured. She spoke little English but glowed with joy.

'Charlie is wonderful!' she said. 'He has the hands of an angel. You will do well. We are so lucky, aren't we?'

Aaron remained an object of fascination for the medical fraternity. He appeared, officially this time, in front of a large group of doctors, answering questions and running through his visual and touch tests with Erica Jacobsen like a circus act. The neurologists asked about tingling, numbness, headaches, difficulty with reading. An elderly man with a European accent asked if he had experienced any hallucinations.

'Yes,' said Aaron. 'I came home one day and saw a little girl in my left vision, holding out her hands to me.'

Until then, Aaron had not thought to tell any of his doctors about the apparitions that visited him – ghosts, perhaps, or a strange, vivid symptom of his illness.

The little girl had been waiting for him one night when he got home from a recording session. He saw her as he opened the door and stepped into the hallway. She wasn't anyone he recognised, just a sweet child with blond hair, who stood with her hands cupped as though asking for something. For a moment, Aaron thought she was real until he walked on and the girl disappeared. He was surprised but not unnerved, and in his stressed-out condition she was just one more oddity.

'I saw the little girl again,' he told his neighbour Andi the next time she materialised. She stood in the hallway two or three more times and, although he didn't attach a supernatural meaning to the image, he thought later that she seemed to represent some kind of urgent need, perhaps his own. That might well have been so but medicine, of course, has a less fanciful explanation; drugs, schizophrenia, migraine, epilepsy, blindness and damage to certain parts of the brain can all cause hallucinations. Aaron's tumour compressed the area of his brain that controls spatio-visual coordination, so that he bumped into objects that fell within his blind spot and filled in other images that weren't there.

The British neuroscientist V.S. Ramachandran suggests in his book *Phantoms in the Brain* that 'bizarre visual hallucinations are simply an exaggerated version of the processes that occur in your brain and mine every time we let our imagination run free. Somewhere in the confused welter of interconnecting forward and backward pathways is the interface between vision and imagination . . . To overstate the argument deliberately, perhaps we are hallucinating all the time and what we call perception is arrived at by simply determining which hallucination best conforms to the current sensory input. But if . . . the brain does not receive confirming visual stimuli, it is free simply to make up its own reality.'

Ramachandran notes that a surprising number of people with visual handicaps in one study of hallucinations reported seeing children. But Aaron's visitations did not end with the little girl. Later they would become even more elaborate and surreal. They seemed to open a window into the workings of his brain and even into the workings of the universe.

PART TWO

PART TWO

'We are not interested in the fact that the brain has the consistency of cold porridge.'

Alan Turing

12

PIONEERS

Endoscopic brain surgery is at the frontier of modern medicine: neurosurgery at its most refined and its most distant from the gory past. In the opinion of Mitch Berger, the chairman of neurological surgery at the University of California in San Francisco, 'Charlie Teo is the most experienced endoscopic neurosurgeon in the world. Very few people in medicine are innovators. Charlie developed the field of modern endoscopy. He goes to meetings and people's jaws drop: how is this possible?' Bernard Kwok, head of neurosurgery at Prince of Wales, has a name for Charlie's specialty – tumours that might be low-grade and curable but are deep in the brain and hard to access except by endoscopy – he calls them 'Teo-omas'.

Charlie is by no means the only surgeon using endoscopy but he performs with authority and can claim better-than-average results. He explained the procedure during an operation at Prince of Wales Private Hospital on a seven-year-old boy who had a colloid cyst blocking the passage between the ventricles in the centre of his brain. The build-up of spinal fluid caused by the tiny low-grade tumour was giving him headaches but, more seriously, if left untreated the pressure from the fluid could have caused sudden death.

'Normally this would be major surgery,' Charlie said, contrasting his way with the 'old' way. 'It could take four hours. Part of the skull would be removed and you'd have to go between the two halves of the brain. It's one of the most common causes of medico-legal action because it's such a dangerous part of the brain.'

Sometimes he would approach these gelatinous growths through a nostril or an incision under the eyebrow. This time he made a three-centimetre cut on the boy's scalp, drilled a pencil-width hole and inserted the endoscope – a flexible microscope on a fine metal probe – between the brain fibres and into the third ventricle, which, in a small child, is a narrow space. Rather than watching his hands, Charlie followed the progress of the endoscope through the brain's pink tunnels on a monitor. The cyst showed up like a pearl in the magnified image. Charlie held the endoscope, maintaining a precise angle of entry, while his assisting neurosurgeon grabbed the cyst with tiny pincers. Pieces kept breaking off and he lost his hold. For a whole minute, the cyst blocked the fine instrument and irrigating fluid flooded the brain. The patient's blood pressure rose and his heartbeat faltered. Then the cyst moved. The almost bloodless operation had taken less than an hour. Charlie watched the boy's eyes for cognitive ill effects as he regained consciousness but there were none. He went home the next morning.

Endoscopy is suitable only for a small range of hard-to-reach tumours and Aaron's was not among them. A large, bloody growth surrounded by solid brain tissue, it needed a wider opening that gave clear access and direct vision. But Charlie would still use his signature techniques. He would shave a small patch of Aaron's scalp, make a relatively short incision and remove a tiny cup of bone. His way carries its own risks: limited access and intricate manoeuvres are not for every doctor or every patient. Over the years, though, he has demonstrated that his patients suffer minimal trauma and recover quickly; just waking up with hair rather than a bandaged head is good for the spirit.

In the brief history of his specialty, Charlie belongs to a line of mavericks. The man who performed the first modern brain surgery was William Macewen, the chairman of surgery at Glasgow University in the late nineteenth century. A famous story about Macewen tells of how he once found himself sharing a train compartment with two women and a drunk who refused to be quiet. Macewen placed his large hands around the man's head and dislocated his jaw. On approaching his destination, he reached out and reset the silent man's bones.

Macewen was a student of Joseph Lister, the pioneer of anti-sepsis, which combined with anaesthesia to advance the possibilities for surgery in the late nineteenth century. At the time, doctors had the difficulty of calculating where to open the skull without the benefit of X-rays. There was, as well, a taboo attached to the very idea of tampering with the brain. A Scottish outsider in the English medical establishment, Macewen was disliked by many of his colleagues for his stubborn, independent nature and sarcastic humour. In 1879, he operated on a fourteen-year-old girl who had a swelling over her left eye and suffered convulsions of the right side of her face and right arm. By simple observation he deduced the site of her problem, cut a hole in her skull with a circular saw and removed a swelling on the covering membrane of her brain. She made a full recovery. The doctor was convinced that surgery could also cure brain tumours, believed by most of the medical profession to be incurable. He was, however, overtaken.

A 25-year-old Scottish farmer, his name recorded only as Henderson, was the first person to submit to surgery for a brain tumour, in November 1884. He was suffering from headaches, convulsive attacks, weakness in his left hand and a limp in his left leg. His doctor had treated him with mustard-plasters on the head and neck, leaving his skin inflamed and blistered. Alexander Hughes Bennett, a neurologist at the National Hospital in London, was certain the man had a brain tumour, and that he could identify its precise location and remove it. It was understood by that time that each hemisphere of the brain controlled the opposite side of the body. By analysing which parts of the man's body were disabled, Bennett concluded the tumour was about five centimetres in diameter and situated in the centre right of the brain. The patient clung to him and said, 'I'll thank you no matter what happens. I'll always thank you.'

The surgery was executed reluctantly by Lister's nephew and assistant at King's College Hospital, Rickman Godlee, a young man who, though a good technician, was completely inexperienced in brain surgery. In a makeshift theatre sterilised with carbolic acid, Godlee dipped his scalpel into carbolic and made two long intersecting incisions. An assistant sponged the blood, clamped the spurting blood vessels and folded back the four flaps of skin. Bennett's shaking hand pointed to the piece of skull that needed removal and Godlee took up his trepan, a serrated saw bent into a circle, and turned its handle to carve a small round section out of the bone. A cut into the underlying membrane caused the brain to bulge but there was no sign of a tumour.

Godlee trepanned a second overlapping hole, then a third. He used a chisel and hammer to chip away splinters of bone and connect the three openings into a large triangle.

Still there was no tumour. To find out if the growth lay deeper, Godlee had to step over the forbidden line and slice into the brain itself. The tissue parted and a centimetre in he could see a hard, round lump like a pigeon's egg. He heated a metal spatula over a flame, bent it into a spoon shape, and pried the tumour from the brain. But when he tried to scoop it out with his forefinger it tore, and then the bleeding began. As the surgeon scraped away at the remaining tumour, blood flowed too fast for the sponges the nurse handed him. Without knowing what damage it would cause, he heated his galvanocautery – a simple instrument for sealing blood vessels – and placed it into the cavity left by the tumour. The hot metal sizzled against wet tissue. The bleeding stopped.

Within days, Henderson was mentally active and free of the headaches and convulsions. He could use his left leg, though his left arm was paralysed. But, a month after the operation, he died. Neither the tumour nor the surgery was directly to blame. An infection had led to meningitis, perhaps carried by the sponges or by the pre-operative cleansing with carbolic that had washed bacteria into the incision from the sores on his head. Even so, the two doctors had proved that brain surgery was possible and effective. The basic procedure they followed, though more pre-carious, was not radically different from the surgery practised today by neurosurgeons such as Charlie Teo.

It was an American doctor, Harvey Cushing, who in the early twentieth century developed neurosurgery into a specialty with an image of intellectual charisma. As a recent account by an American doctor, Christopher J. Wahl, explains, 'within thirty years [he] had taken surgery on the brain from a nearly unanimously fatal act of desperation to a legitimate practice in American medicine'. Cushing was famous for his compassionate, holistic care for patients combined with a tendency to be demanding, sarcastic and bad-tempered, refusing to admit mistakes or allow anyone else to share his limelight, and sometimes bringing student nurses to tears in the operating theatre. By the end of his career, he had reduced the mortality rate for brain tumour operations from ninety to eight per cent.

The next leap forward came with microsurgery, which gave neurosurgeons the means to cut and mend the brain's narrow corrugations, minute blood vessels and hidden lesions. One of the leaders was Gazi Yasargil, named 'Man of the Century 1950–1999' by the international Congress of Neurological Surgeons. Born in 1925 in Turkey, he studied at the University of Vermont in Burlington, where micro-vascular surgery was developed in the late 1950s. He began applying the new techniques and instruments to reconstructing brain arteries in animals.

That old problem, the fragility of the brain's blood vessels, hindered his work until he used another new tool – bipolar coagulation technology. Yasargil adapted the bipolar – a two-pronged forceps heated by an electric current that burns shut the tiniest vessels – into an essential implement for neurosurgeons. But the most revolutionary piece of equipment he developed was the floating microscope, a lens that hung over the patient, gave five- to ten-times magnification, and could be manipulated with an electromagnetic mouth switch that left the hands free. Yasargil's microscope enabled him to perform the first cerebral vascular bypass operation in 1967 and became standard in operating theatres.

After working for most of his career in Zurich, Yasargil retired in 1993 and became professor of neurosurgery at the University of Arkansas for Medical Sciences. The chairman of the department, Ossama Al-Mefty, described him as exemplifying 'the operative neurosurgeon, in whom a brilliant mind and a developed soul guide gifted hands'. This was the department that also hired Charlie Teo as assistant professor of neurosurgery in 1994. The two men worked for several years as partners, often operating together. Yasargil has practised into his eighties, with surgical courage and steadiness of hand. Charlie learned a sustaining lesson from the man who was in many ways a kindred spirit.

'He never sat down and taught me to do things, but he taught me that it can be done. The sky's the limit. He taught me not to accept dogma as a given. If that tumour has been classified as inoperable, don't accept that. It's not inoperable. If you can do it, you can do it. I saw him take out inoperable tumours and I thought, "Hang on, if he can do that I can probably do it." I was always like that anyway, but it gave me more courage to keep trying new things.'

It would be wrong to draw too neat a likeness between the two men, but they often sound like one mind speaking with different voices. Yasargil has said in *Neurosurgery* journal: 'I contrive to help my patients as long as they will accept surgical treatment. There is no area in the CNS [central nervous system] that cannot be accessed in a proper manner with removal of the lesion and an acceptable outcome.' He also insists: 'Our role is to hold the door open, so that hope and optimism may enter, and to psychologically invigorate and sustain the patients throughout the duration of their illness.'

In the pattern of neurosurgical pioneers, Yasargil has critics as well as devotees. A former student wrote that his early results were met with rejection, disbelief and jealousy among the establishment because they were dramatically better than previous reports. Yasargil is said to be tough and arrogant, and was not widely liked among the faculty in Little Rock when Charlie was there. Like Cushing, he has a fierce temper, doesn't tolerate mistakes and is quick to dismiss students and surgeons. He is frugal with compliments but once told a medical instrument maker in Germany that Charlie was the best neurosurgeon he had ever seen. Charlie calls Yasargil 'a legend'.

Mitch Berger, Charlie's peer at the University of California, puts the Australian in the same class as Yasargil. 'He is an innovator in technique and he is also a master technician. I've seen him operate. There are people who are technically proficient and solid, but his hands are incredible, the way he handles instruments. He belongs in an elite of less than one or two per cent in the world.' Charlie, he says, 'is down to earth, ethical, phenomenal in his compassion. Every time I've seen him in conversation about patient care it's not about him, it's about the patient. A lot of people try to sell you things; they tell you they're the best in the field. Charlie has always maintained a cool, logical head. You have to go out and be aggressive if you are going to do new things. He's never had the reputation of a cowboy in America . . . And it's not as if I'm even friendly with the guy.'

Charlie hopes the next generation of neurosurgeons will take his minimally invasive methods into the mainstream. Even now, a few younger surgeons are beginning to make him look conservative. He has been doing endoscopic surgery on brain tumours through the nose for fifteen years, but has always stopped at the carotid artery – the major vessel in the neck – and made a more conventional approach. A young neurosurgeon from Pittsburgh, Amin Kassam, who attended one of Charlie's meetings on keyhole surgery at the University of New South

Wales in 2005, is daring to take tumours involving the carotid through the nose. In time he might even claim the 'I'm not quite sure you can believe this guy' mantle.

Though Charlie's critics will never agree, the performance of the next generation of neurosurgeons could push him into the ranks of the establishment. It hasn't happened yet. Another American, Dan Kelly, a professor at the University of California Los Angeles, came to Sydney as a student in 1989 and met Charlie when he was still a volatile young registrar. As an admirer of his technical skills and frontier-pushing techniques, Kelly also came back for the keyhole symposium in 2005.

'Charlie hasn't changed much,' he said then. 'He's a rebel with a cause.'

13

STOLEN BLOOD

Geoffrey Parker, the neuroradiologist at Royal Prince Alfred Hospital, had returned from his holiday, and Charlie was depending on him to make his own job less dangerous by reducing the bloodiness of Aaron's tumour. Parker would see Aaron on the morning of Wednesday 15 August 2001 and Charlie would operate within forty-eight hours of the embolisation. If Aaron's brain swelled uncontrollably during the first procedure, Royal Prince Alfred would have another neurosurgery team ready to do an emergency operation, so there was still a chance that Charlie would not be in charge.

Aaron had several tasks to face, some unpleasant but necessary. He had asked David Wansbrough to preside at his funeral service if that was how the story ended, and David brought in a lawyer to help Aaron complete his will. With few material possessions – no real estate, no car, only his piano – his companies never-theless had to be settled. He wanted to sum up all the serious thinking he had done in a few words for *Australian Story*. Sitting alone under the lamplight, he wrote:

> Just as a game, tell yourself that you could be six weeks from the end of your life right now. You could be. Suddenly a lot of complicated things become very simple. You can forget about all the things that revolve around you and start focusing on the reason you were given this life in the first place. Be absolutely definitive. Find what it is that binds you to this life, because we're given the opportunity to work on that every day. And then one day, suddenly, it can all be taken away.

Later that night, Aaron crept past the sleeping patients to his piano room. He needed to express his emotions through music. Rachmaninov's beauty didn't suit the moment. Instead he chose the difficult *Evryali* – 'the sun beating a path across the sky' – by the twentieth-century Greek composer Yannis Xenakis. The sound was fast, harsh and slightly deranged but underpinned by a mathematical harmony that Xenakis also employed as assistant to the great modernist architect Le Corbusier. There was a debate in the music world about whether it was possible to play the piece as written. The intensity was both a challenge and a release – a yell from the soul.

Aaron played the eight-minute *Evryali* straight through with the volume muted, 'to get me in the mood for surgery', and at the same time recorded it into the piano. He wanted the television crew to film the instrument playing it back digitally, the keys banging down like a mad electronic pianola with an invisible player.

At Royal Prince Alfred the next morning, Geoffrey Parker was ready, wearing a surgical gown and a skiing tan. He had known Charlie Teo when he was a neurosurgical registrar and considered him a gifted surgeon. However, it was rare for Charlie to send him a patient. Most of Parker's work was on blood vessels in the central nervous system rather than in tumours, interpreting X-rays and doing procedures such as embolisation using X-ray guidance. Tumours only came to Parker for embolisation when they had what he called 'a very brisk blood supply'. Usually they were meningiomas, which arose from the membranes covering the brain rather than inside the brain itself. But it wasn't always possible to tell what kind of tumour a patient had until surgery, and Aaron's was so large and pushing so deeply into the brain that its origin was not at all obvious.

He studied the scans and saw 'a rather alarming tumour, like a funny, lobulated cauliflower'. He hoped it had its own blood supply, separate from the brain's. He could then squirt PVA particles – plastic granules like very fine sand – into some of the blood vessels through a fine plastic tube called a catheter, which would make the larger vessels and their tiny branches shut down, shrinking or even liquefying the tumour. When Charlie operated, he would have to cut fewer vessels, resulting in less blood loss and faster surgery. Aaron's chance of 'doing well' would be much improved. Parker likened the difference to a plumber who was trying to fix a pipe at the bottom of a hole: it was much easier if the water was turned off.

Parker approached the brain with a catheter inserted way down in the groin, into the large femoral artery that emerged from the trunk and ran down the leg. To make such a journey, the catheter had to be one hundred and eighty centimetres long with a guide wire running through it that could turn corners into the narrower blood vessels. Parker manipulated the catheter up the highway of arteries with his hands and watched its progress on a screen. At best, the insertion of a catheter carried a one-in-five-hundred risk of forming a blood clot that could cause a stroke and a one-in-two-hundred risk of a minor stroke with no after effects. But in a case like Aaron's, it had a greater chance of saving his life.

The first step was to give Aaron an angiogram and identify the blood vessels feeding his tumour. He was laid out on a table and injected with a local anaesthetic near the top of his leg. A gowned and masked Parker pushed the catheter into his groin through a syringe and it appeared like a speeding worm on the X-ray screen as it raced up his body. Blood vessels have no sensation, so Aaron was oblivious until Parker removed the guide wire from the catheter and caused a rush of heat with an injection of dye that would show up as a river system on his brain images.

Parker instantly disliked what the X-rays revealed.

'The problem here is that all these vessels we're showing so far supply the normal brain and you can't embolise them; you can't block off the blood supply.'

He thought the tumour was most likely a low-grade meningioma, but it had formed a complex network of parasitised blood vessels from the brain. If Parker injected PVA into them, they would carry it straight to the brain and cause Aaron to have a stroke. Parker phoned Charlie as he examined the images and explained in detail which arteries and veins were involved. Bottom line: there would be no embolisation. Charlie was on his own.

Aaron was still lying down when Parker told him the bad news. The doctor kept it simple and clear. 'On the upside,' he added, 'it is not the most richly supplied one of these we've ever seen and the blood supply is coming from underneath and at the back. So Charlie thinks he can take most of that as he comes in and approaches the tumour, which is a good thing.'

'That's good, okay,' Aaron said.

Charlie scheduled the operation for early the next morning, fortuitously a Thursday when he was always in the public hospital. He was used to reeling off all the things that could go wrong during surgery, but usually he knew deep down that things would go well. When he had to tell a patient that things were looking really, really bad, it was hard to sound even more serious than usual. Aaron's risk of dying on the operating table had just risen to between ten and fifteen per cent.

Aaron accepted Charlie's pronouncements readily, almost glibly, and didn't ask for a second opinion. Even patients who travelled from overseas, knowing they wanted Charlie's expertise, often expressed some doubt or apprehension, which he thought was healthy. But Aaron seemed to have complete confidence in him. Charlie thought for a moment that Aaron's tumour might have caused a medical syndrome known as *la belle indifférence*, where sufferers show a cool lack of response to the worst news. Told that their family had been slaughtered, they might say, 'Okay.' It was the brain's coping mechanism and sometimes tumours could set it off. But Charlie knew Aaron's tumour wasn't in a place that would have that effect, and he wondered why he had not seen the young man go through the usual phases of denial, anger, acceptance and projection as he considered his predicament. Most people experienced the defensive sequence over days if not hours. But Aaron had not been angry, nor had he tried to blame anyone else. He had not been in denial, except for that first burst of impatience when he wanted to get back to recording his album. Maybe he had dealt privately with his emotions. Whatever the case, he certainly wasn't a typical patient.

Charlie spelled out again the reason embolisation had been impossible and that it would make the operation trickier. He raised another problem. Aaron's tumour sat on top of the vein of Galen, a major blood vessel named after a major figure in early Western medicine, which drained the blood from all the deep structures of the brain. The walls of the vein were extremely thin and delicate, and the slightest bump could tear them, causing unstoppable bleeding and instant death. The X-rays had shown that the tumour was actually wrapped around the vein, compressing and deforming it. Charlie would try to identify the vein before he damaged it. If the tumour had invaded it, he would have to leave some of the growth behind and deal with it later. If the tumour peeled off neatly, that would be great, but if he hit the vein before seeing it, 'that would be very bad'.

Charlie had brought along Peter Nakaji, a young American neurosurgeon who was at Prince of Wales on a fellowship. Aaron's would be his last operation with Charlie before flying back to California.

'So, you're going to have the A-team helping you tomorrow,' Charlie told Aaron. 'You'll be having a good old sleep, that's all.'

'I've got plenty to achieve, I think, so there's got to be a purpose.'

'We'll get going first thing in the morning and we'll see you after the operation. Good luck.'

Charlie reached out and shook Aaron's hand. Both men smiled. Then Charlie tucked his hands back in the pockets of his monogrammed white coat and moved on to his other patients. The next time he saw Aaron, he would be peering inside his head.

Gail stayed by her son's side. There had been no deep and meaningful conversations. Most of their talk was about the practicalities of treatment, meals, laundry, visitors. Questions of life and death and love were almost impossible to put into words. Now they tossed them lightly into the air.

Gail leaned down and said, 'I have complete faith in the A-team.'

'I'll just have a nice little sleep tomorrow and if I meet Saint Peter at the gates I'll stay away from the light. Isn't that the rule?' Aaron squeezed out a laugh.

'I love you heaps,' Gail said. 'I'll be praying for you. We're fighters. We've been through a lot in our lives and we'll get through this.'

She wrapped him in hugs and kisses, and her parents stepped in to give him more. For now, that was all they could do.

14

THE MIND BOMB

After a long search on the morning of Aaron McMillan's surgery, Charlie Teo eventually found his lucky socks amid the dirty washing. They were worn threadbare in places but the joke was still legible: *World's greatest fuck*.

The night before, he and his wife had turned over the implications of the case. Charlie thrived on stress, and Genevieve was always impressed by how he could come home from a death-defying day and transform into a devoted father. It was only after a patient died that the house felt a little bleaker. This time, though, Genevieve thought Charlie was risking his career, and couldn't believe he was allowing a television crew to film an operation with such an uncertain outcome.

'Genevieve, we've got to accept the good with the bad,' Charlie told her. 'We've had good press and maybe my colleagues will leave me alone if they see me fall flat on my face. Maybe that's what they want to see. I'll give it to them and then they'll leave me alone.'

Aaron was also preparing himself for the challenge. Overnight, in the hospital's brief quietness, he had reaffirmed his determination to live and had slept for a few hours. In the dark hours of the morning, he went to the piano and played his Rachmaninov prelude one more time, just for himself, lingering on the last exquisite chord.

His mother and father, David Wansbrough and Peter Crisp hurried in at around 6 am, trying to hide their anxiety. They kissed Aaron and wished him good luck and went to find distraction in breakfast.

Aaron felt no fear as he was trundled through the fluorescent-lit corridors. He had farewelled the nurses and his old roommate Arnold and all the patients he'd come to know from wandering the ward and playing the piano.

Down on the first floor, in the labyrinth of theatres, he met a new team of anaesthetists and nurses who would undertake the preparations for surgery. All he knew was the sound of objects being pulled off shelves, alien clanks, rustles, beeps, pumping air and voices directed not at him. A scramble to find a post-operative bed in intensive care slowed things down again.

It was a relief when Teigan, the ABC sound recordist, loomed above him wearing a silly blue surgical cap and a grin. 'Howdy,' she said. Aaron laughed. She looked ready to perform the operation herself. Ben and Steve, the producer and cameraman, were there in blue, too, and their ease buoyed his spirits.

Aaron didn't know that Teigan and Steve had sat down with a six-pack of beer the night before to talk about the etiquette of filming the operation and talking to his family, especially if things went badly. They met again to watch the sun rise and cheer, 'Fuck the cosmos!' before leaving for the hospital. They had taken their catchcry from one of several poems David Wansbrough wrote about Aaron, which ended:

It is all for the greater glory of God.

If that is so, and God wants this glory
then fuck God, fuck the Cosmos . . .
This boy whose life seemed such a gift
must live!

The delicate process of sinking Aaron into unconsciousness took almost two hours. It began when the anaesthetist, Richard Connolly, injected a sedative into his left hand.

'We're just going to make you a bit light-headed here. You probably won't remember much after this,' he said.

'I'm coming back,' said Aaron. 'I love this world. I'll be here.'

He smiled serenely as the drug began to work. Connolly held an oxygen mask over his face and asked, 'How are you going, Aaron? Still with us, mate?' There was no answer.

Oddly, considering it is the organ that is the centre of the body's sensations, the brain itself feels no pain. Neurosurgeons can keep their patients awake if, for example, they are operating close to the area for speech, and need to hear if the ability to talk is affected when they touch a certain spot. They can prod inside an epileptic's brain and ask how it feels. But Aaron's would sleep through his operation, his body would be paralysed and a ventilator would breathe for him. Tubes and catheters would carry fluids in and out. Machines would monitor his heart and circulation. He would retain no memories of the meddling inside his head.

*

Charlie strode through the double doors into Theatre A3 at 9.30 am and chucked his motorcycle helmet in a corner. He was expecting to operate for about eight hours if all went well, maybe more if there were complications. By this stage he still calculated Aaron's risk of death during surgery at ten to fifteen per cent. But he went in, as always, planning to win.

His team that day was a mixture of hand-picked registrars, colleagues and strangers – some friends and one or two antagonists. He had passed through the hospital the day before and warned the nurses they would be working on his most challenging operation yet.

Judith McKenzie had been a theatre nurse at Prince of Wales for sixteen years, specialising in neurosurgery. When she arrived that morning and saw Aaron's scans lit up on the wall showing the white nuclear mushroom cloud, she gasped, 'Oh no.' But she'd worked with Charlie Teo before and knew he was good. She wasn't apprehensive as she helped to organise the instruments she would hand to the anaesthetic nurse and scrub nurse at his side.

Charlie's primary assistant was David Kadrian, a keen young registrar just three years out of university. This was his first neurosurgical case. Peter Nakaji, the visiting American fellow, was preparing to fly home the next day; he would join them for the first stage of the operation then return again after a few hours. Optimistically, Charlie and Genevieve were throwing him a farewell party at their house that night. Others, such as Erica Jacobsen, the registrar who had cared for Aaron, would come in to watch and help for short stints. Only Charlie would be there without a break for as long as it took.

'Let's have some music!' he shouted as though a party was about to begin. One of the nurses slid a CD into the tinny player.

Charlie's favourite bands and singers – Elvis Presley, John Denver, Abba and a few others – accompanied most of his operations. Like many surgeons, he concentrated better with music in the background, except in moments of emergency. As with patients, the right music can lower a surgeon's blood pressure and pulse rate. It also filters out extraneous thoughts and sounds. Some choose classical or jazz, and one surgeon at Prince of Wales prefers rap. Others insist on silence. Whatever their personal tastes, Charlie's staff learned to put up with, and even appreciate, his golden oldies and his bursts of song. It made their long days less wearing. No one realised as Elvis rocked and crooned that day, 16 August 2001, that it was the anniversary of his death in 1977, the year Aaron was born. It was a long time to have been dead; not so long to have lived.

Charlie began as he always did by bringing out a comb and disposable razor to shave a patch at the back of Aaron's scalp. An offsider could have done it but Charlie liked setting the patient up, positioning him and making sure the incision was in the right spot. Sometimes that could be the difference between an operable and an inoperable tumour. He kept the shaved area small because patients felt better if they still had hair when they woke up. Like an old-fashioned barber, he combed a knife-sharp part through the wet curls and scraped them away.

Face down, his head gripped by a clamp, painted with iodine and wrapped in adhesive plastic, his body bundled in blankets and topped with a sterile green sheet, Aaron no longer resembled a person. Only the circle of yellowed skin on his scalp was exposed.

Scrubbed and tied into a green gown, blue cap, white paper mask, clear goggles and skin-tight latex gloves, with his lucky socks hidden inside wooden-soled clogs, Charlie was hardly recognisable either.

The room was kept at a steady seventeen degrees. A surgical team could easily overheat during the intensity of a long operation, so the cool air kept them comfortable and dry and unlikely to spread germs, which can travel through a sweaty glove. For anyone else, the operating theatre was an icebox.

Blood started to flow the moment Charlie made the first cut using his 'knife and fork', a scalpel and forceps used to hold back the layers of scalp, which are thicker and fleshier than they feel when stretched over bone. With a whining power drill, he pierced holes and removed a piece of Aaron's skull the size of a fifty-cent coin, spitting splinters of bone across the room like coconut shavings. Most neurosurgeons would give themselves more working room with a bigger craniotomy, but Charlie was convinced that almost any operation could be done through a narrower opening.

One more cut was needed to penetrate the dura mater (the beautifully named 'tough mother'), a fibrous white membrane that is the brain's last layer of protection. Charlie noted that the dura, which usually lay flat and slack, was tense from the pressure beneath. There it was: Aaron's poor inflamed brain, crammed into its shell.

In his right hand, Charlie held a bipolar coagulation forceps to shut off blood vessels with heat and sometimes a puff of smoke. It also served, like chopsticks, to pick up, separate, stretch and pull tissues. In his left hand he held a micro-sucker, a gentler version of the instrument used by dentists to remove saliva from the mouth. It kept his view clear by draining the cavity of blood as well as the irrigation fluid pumped in almost constantly by the scrub nurse to keep the brain alive. Used clumsily, however, the micro-sucker could also remove brain tissue and damage or kill a patient.

At different times a nurse would hand him grabbing forceps,

scissors and dissectors, but mostly he would probe and push the tissues with the bipolar and sucker. To an outsider he might as well have been reaching down a narrow drainpipe to dismantle a bomb with knitting needles.

Aaron's tumour wasn't immediately visible. The grey matter, a term we commonly use for the brain as a whole, forms only a few millimetres of the wrinkled surface, and Charlie usually worked in the white matter below it. But he knew he couldn't cut through the tissue in that area, so he carefully parted the two hemispheres along the dividing membrane called the falx. He wouldn't even risk damage by using metal retractors to widen the opening.

About two centimetres in he could see the denser off-white matter of the tumour. 'That's good,' he thought. It was not as deep in as he had feared and it had taken him only half an hour to reach it. As suspected, it seemed to be growing from the falx. That was good, too, better than growing out of the brain tissue.

With the lights dimmed, he rolled in the big overhead micro-scope with its own bright headlight, five hundred thousand dollars' worth of equipment that enabled to him to keep his head up while looking straight down into Aaron's brain. He began removing the tumour, easing it away and pulling it out, fragment by tiny fragment. He could see major blood vessels such as the vein of Galen, as thick as his little finger, and knew it would be fatal to hit them, but it was impossible to avoid the hundreds of micro-vessels running through the tumour.

Within ten minutes he was in trouble. It might take fifteen seconds to extract a skerrick of tumour but then he had to spend another two minutes staunching the blood.

'It just keeps welling up on me,' he said.

Blood flowed out through the sucker into clear canisters

and back in, as it was needed, from big bags controlled by the anaesthetist.

Charlie persevered but after four or five hours he began to worry.

'Shit,' he said. 'I should be making more progress than this.'

If he stepped back and looked with his naked eye, he seemed to have achieved nothing, and now he could barely get access to the tumour. The more he removed, the more the brain swelled, and it had begun to push out of the craniotomy. He'd seen that before and if it didn't improve, the only way to treat it was to resect some of the brain so he could get back to the tumour. Some frontal tumours cause the brain to mushroom and part of the frontal lobe can be removed with minimal consequences. Scary though it sounds, it is possible to cut eight centimetres back and lop off the frontal lobe on one side. Although that part of the brain controls functions such as eye movement, continence, parts of the personality, memory storage and some coordination of movement, when one half stops working, the other can do the whole job.

But this was very different. Not only was the tumour bloody and in a delicate area, but any damage would most likely end Aaron's career. And if he couldn't read music and play the piano, he might as well not be alive.

Another of Charlie's patients, with a different type of tumour in the same area, came out of his operation with his eye–hand coordination disrupted. He could no longer place a telephone receiver back on its cradle with his left hand. Others were left hemiplegic, or paralysed down one side, from simpler operations on similar tumours. One patient was fully functional except for a useless eye. So Charlie decided to try everything to reduce the swelling before cutting Aaron's brain.

He used a needle to withdraw spinal fluid from the left ventricle, until there was no fluid left and the space in the ventricle had collapsed from the pressure. He then had the anaesthetist use two different intravenous drugs to dehydrate the brain. He tilted the bed so that Aaron's head was higher than his feet, making the blood flow away from his brain. Charlie had to stand on a stool to continue operating.

The anaesthetist tried hyperventilation, getting the machine to breathe faster and faster so that there was more oxygen and less carbon dioxide in Aaron's lungs.

Then they brought out the barbiturate thiopentone – the big gun according to Charlie – which decreases the brain's metabolic need and so reduces the blood supply and, in theory, the swelling. Charlie had only used the drug a few times and considered it a last resort.

Nothing worked.

After six hours, Charlie should have had the tumour out and been preparing to close up. But there he was with Aaron's brain bulging out of the hole in his skull and blood gushing up at him. It was time to warn his family that things were going to be as bad as Charlie had feared, and maybe worse. He was about to cut into Aaron's brain to try to save his life.

Around 3 pm, Charlie sent David Kadrian out to find Gail Puckett and give her the news.

15

MOTHER AND SON

Gail had set her alarm for 4.30 am and woken at three. As she drove from her parents' house through the chilled grey morning, a billboard caught her eye. It showed a photograph of the Whitsunday Islands and the lure *Cancel next week*. Hunched over the wheel at a red light, she thought, 'Please, God, cancel this day. Just this day will be enough, thank you very much.'

She said a brief goodbye to Aaron and after a tense breakfast returned to the ward to send him off properly. But his bed was empty. He had been wheeled away to the operating theatre just after seven o'clock. In a panic, Gail wondered if she would see her son again. She planned to spend the day alone. Her spirituality had sedimentary layers from her Catholic upbringing, years of Buddhist meditation, more recent studies in anthroposophy and New Age smatterings. She believed that while his physical body was under anaesthetic, his 'finer bodies' – the spiritual, the emotional and the inner life force – would disperse and be unprotected. Her job was to hold him in her thoughts and protect his energy. She was also drawn back into her family's traditions. She had persuaded her parents to stay at home and they had each agreed to repeat a prayer for him every hour – Gail on the hour, Frank and Marjorie on the half-hour – during his surgery.

For the first time since the whirlwind of Aaron's illness began, Gail had time to go into the solid old Catholic Church of the Sacred Heart on a busy street near the hospital. She sat for a while at the back, then moved to a smaller chapel at one side where a marble statue of a serene Mary held her curly-haired baby son. Gail had always felt a strong connection with Christianity's mother figure and now, praying for her own son, she was conscious of their shared pain. In her pocket she had a recent photograph of Aaron sitting in a chair at his grandmother's house, his hands large in the foreground. She took it out and placed her hand on his hand.

'There,' she thought, 'I've got you. You're not going anywhere.'

She prayed and bargained fiercely for her son's life, and for her own ability to cope if she had to let him go or had to take him home disabled in a wheelchair. With Aaron's photograph in one hand and a Catholic prayer card in the other, bathed in blue and gold light from the stained-glass windows, she stayed there for three hours.

'My prayer,' she said, 'is that Aaron has a miraculously successful operation with positive outcomes, and that in his heart and his whole inner being he has change to his whole life after his operation. I know there are millions of children dying every day . . . and I've managed to have this child for twenty-four years, so I should consider myself lucky and I don't dare to presume what plans You have for Aaron. I'm not saying give him to me just so I can be satisfied as a mother when You have thousands of mothers in this world who are losing children every day. How dare I? But he needs to lead his life; he hasn't had a chance to experience life and he has so much to give.'

At lunchtime she walked back out into the glare and rumble of the street, looking for a place to eat though she had no appetite. It was as if time had stopped. She could see every freckle on strangers' faces. All their hurry and worry seemed pointless. They should enjoy being alive.

Reluctantly, Gail returned to the hospital, where friends had transformed Aaron's piano into a makeshift altar, with flowers, photographs and sheet music. Aaron's unfinished CD played softly in the background. Brian was among the small group meditating and praying. He was both insider and outsider. As a father, he would not take Aaron's loss lightly. Yet, he easily stepped back into Buddhist meditation to clear his mind. When David Kadrian appeared with his report from the operating theatre just after three o'clock, Brian continued to breathe evenly and began to repeat, 'May the swelling decrease; may the surgeon have the opportunity to get to the tumour.' He thought, 'It's okay, whatever the outcome. If Aaron has decided to go on, we give thanks for the wonderful comet that's come down into our universe briefly and passed off like Mozart and Keats and Jesus. Their role was a brief one but a very powerful one.' He found himself in a relaxed and even blissful state of acceptance.

Gail ran to the bathroom and splashed her face with water as she prepared for the next round. She withdrew again to the bare room where Aaron had often lain alone staring up at the night sky. Kneeling on a rubber cushion, she watched the day fade and focused again on the bond with her son. There was a time, twenty years before, when he could have lost her. Driving him to kindergarten, she had nosed her old Datsun onto a six-lane highway just as the traffic lights were changing. As she crossed the peak-hour traffic, another car emerged from behind a truck and slammed into hers. The Datsun rolled twice before landing back on its wheels. Gail was knocked unconscious with her foot pressed down on the accelerator. The car sped off the road, into an open garage and up the rear of a Mini Minor. A worried stranger peered in the window and found Aaron in the front passenger seat, unbruised and seemingly unshaken.

Gail was taken to hospital and released that day, but in her brush with mortality she heard the heavenly choirs people had told her about. At that moment, she knew she could have broken her connection with the world. Since then, she had read about near-death experiences and the beckoning light that many people saw. During operations, some patients felt they floated away from their body and didn't want to return. Her own father, undergoing a heart bypass, had seen himself led away by a Christ-child figure to a room full of white-haired men who said, 'What are you doing here? It's not your time.'

Absorbed in her thoughts, Gail gradually became aware of a crying baby in the hospital ward. Curiosity and some inner need drove her out of the room to find that a nurse with a new baby was visiting the staff. She asked if she could hold the baby, and a doctor assured the mother, 'Yes, that's all right; she's Aaron's mother.' She returned to her empty room, where she soothed the infant to sleep in her arms and looked out on the darkening suburbs. She needed to clutch the baby and say, 'Right, I'm not letting go of you.' She knew she wasn't being rational, but through another's child she could feel the life force she was mustering for her own.

16

WHAT WOULD
JOHN WAYNE DO?

Charlie was on the verge of panicking at three o'clock that afternoon but he knew that was the worst thing he could do. The bleeding starts, you lose concentration, your hand shakes, you tear blood vessels, there's more bleeding and you've got a disaster. Instead, he had to slow down, step back and think. It took self-control and even cockiness, a confidence that stopped short of blind arrogance. He had to tell himself, 'If I can't do it, no one can.'

Charlie felt proud when he rose to meet a seemingly impossible challenge. When the obvious course might be to give up and begin sucking out brain tissue so the patient would die quickly, he allowed himself a corny thought. What would John Wayne do?

He was a registrar the first time it had happened. A young man came into Emergency with a gunshot wound to the head. The bullet had passed straight through but his carotid artery was severed and blood was gushing. Registrars were often given hopeless cases and Charlie had to handle this one alone. It was chaos from the beginning. Blood everywhere, suckers blocked up, the man's brain pushing out. A tremor started in Charlie's hand. The anaesthetist was nervous, too.

'Do you know what you're doing? Maybe we should call someone in,' he said.

Charlie stopped, took a deep breath, calmed down, and told himself he was invincible. Then he got on with the job. The pause cleared his head and steadied his hand. He stopped the man's bleeding, sewed him up and got him off the table. It was no use: the patient died a couple of days later from the swelling to his brain. But Charlie had done all a surgeon could do.

He'd seen people fail through overconfidence. He thought it was wrong that in Australia there were no distinct sub-specialisations within neurosurgical training and doctors thought they could do everything. But he also applied a human test by asking himself, 'If that was my wife or my child on the table, would I be the right person to do this?'

Everyone in the operating theatre knew there was a crisis. The music was turned off and nobody spoke. The *sound* of a tumour – its texture, the way it went up the sucker – could be just as telling as its appearance, and Charlie's ears were as sensitive as his hands.

When Judith McKenzie's nursing shift ended at four o'clock, the atmosphere was so tense that she didn't dare say goodbye to Peter Nakaji, although she wouldn't see him again. She scrawled a note on a scrap of paper and held it up for him to read: *Peter, it was lovely working with you. Have a great trip.* He nodded silently.

Charlie was glued to the microscope with renewed stamina. He had to reach the tumour through an opening in the brain that was only a centimetre by half a centimetre wide.

Once a neurosurgeon got into trouble, the negative cycle was hard to break. A swollen brain resulted from a reduced blood flow. Less blood going to the brain meant less oxygen, which led to cell damage and further swelling. But if Charlie could break the cycle by decreasing the tumour's bulk, then things should start improving. The brain would shrink back into place, the blood vessels would open up and take in oxygen, and the swelling would continue to subside.

He had scraped at the tumour for eight hours before he reached that turning point. There wasn't an exact moment when he knew the crisis had passed, but over the next hour or so, the job became easier. Even the vein of Galen gave him less trouble than he had feared. The tumour was tightly attached to the big, fragile vessel but Charlie worked slowly and carefully, lifting away specks of bad tissue. Like chipping at an apple with a toothpick, bit by bit, the tumour peeled off without damaging the vein.

It was after eight o'clock when he was satisfied that he had removed every visible tumour cell. He sent Peter Nakaji off to the farewell party his wife was hosting at their home.

'You'd better get out of here or Genevieve will kill me,' he said.

Finally the lights were raised, the music went on and there was relieved chatter as Charlie began the delicate but routine task of closing up. The nurses counted aloud to check that everything inserted into Aaron's head had been removed. The most time-consuming were all the materials used against the geyser of blood. He had lost two of his body's five litres. The final tally: fifty-five cotton balls, one hundred neuropatties, twenty-five swabs, fifteen sponges and twenty haemostats.

The big hole where the tumour had been would never entirely close up because compression had caused some of the brain tissue to die. But it would fill with spinal fluid. Charlie covered it over with a few stitches in the dura, and the scrub nurse handed him the chunk of bone that had been sitting in a dish. It slotted neatly into place and Charlie, like a home handyman, mended Aaron's skull with surgical glue and staples. Finally, using a long, curved needle, he closed the cut with evenly spaced stitches, as unhurried as he had been all day. He would leave a neat scar in the shape of a question mark.

The television crew came back in and Charlie said into the microphone, 'I didn't think he'd stay the distance.' Cheerfully, he added, 'My bladder's telling me to stop pretty soon.'

It was 10.41 pm when Charlie looked at the clock. He had spent more than twelve hours on his feet without a break to eat, drink, urinate or even loosen his muscles. Adrenalin kept him going and it was only when the tension eased that he started to think about his own body. People who worked with him were impressed by his endurance, though a few thought it was macho foolishness.

As Charlie helped unwrap Aaron and detach him from the tangle of technology, he bumped the plastic bag that hung under the patient's head to collect the overflow of fluids. The pale red cocktail tipped down the front of his clothes and he laughed.

'Look. I've pissed myself!'

The television crew had been there all day, filming in short bursts, watching – draped in blankets – from a side room, and carrying occasional, cautious reports to the group camped up in Ward 8. They had agreed with Gail that they would leave if the night had a tragic ending. There would be a sign: if the whole crew appeared after the operation, things weren't too bad; if Ben Cheshire came alone she would steel herself for the worst.

First they interviewed Charlie. 'We've got the whole tumour out. He's still alive. We saved all the big veins down below. I'm very happy, very relieved. It's one of the hardest cases I've ever done. It's going to be very interesting to see how he wakes up.'

Brain surgery patients must be woken gently but quickly. The organ under the knife is also the one shut down by anaesthesia, and the surgeon can only judge the good or ill effects of his work when the brain is fully functioning again. Modern drugs, carefully administered, make the transition seem easy.

Aaron began to float up into consciousness almost as soon as the anaesthetic was withdrawn. Another drug reversed his paralysis. He could hear voices.

'Aaron, hello, mate,' said the anaesthetist, Richard Connolly.

'He's nodding his head. Oh, good,' said Charlie.

'All finished.' Connolly picked up Aaron's right hand. 'Can you give my hand a squeeze? That's not bad. What about over here?' He took Aaron's left hand. 'That's good, excellent. What about your toes? Can you give them a wiggle?'

'Oh, fantastic!' Charlie allowed himself to be excited.

Erica Jacobsen, the registrar who was familiar with Aaron's family, had the enjoyable job of telling them the operation was over and Aaron was awake. But it would be almost another hour before Charlie, his stained operating gear replaced with a white doctor's coat, came down the corridor with the television crew in tow.

'Things went very well,' Charlie told them, reducing the day's anxiety to a happy ending. 'We got it all out and he's awake and moving. He's feeling all right.'

'Awake? You're kidding! Just sounds like Aaron, doesn't it?' Gail threw her arms around her son's doctor and now saviour.

Charlie ran through the risks still remaining. The next twenty-four hours were very important. Aaron could easily develop a blood clot or an infection or seizures. They still didn't know how well he would recover. But, for the moment, Gail was focused on having her son alive.

She rang her parents and then, at last, she was allowed to see Aaron in the post-operative room. He hadn't opened his eyes but David Kadrian assured her he was breathing and his pupils showed that his brain was working normally. She leaned over, hardly daring to touch her son, and whispered, 'Dr Teo did a fantastic job. We're all so proud of you.' He moaned something almost inaudible. He was asking for ice but Gail said, 'Yes, you'll warm up. Everyone's been praying for you. It's okay. Just get through the next twenty-four hours. Everything's going to be fine. Can you hear me?' He groaned. She looked down with pained relief at his battered face – pale, puffy, eyes swollen shut. But inside he was still Aaron.

Everyone was exhausted but no one wanted to go to bed. In the early hours of the morning, Gail and her band of supporters went to the all-night pub across the road where some of the doctors and nurses spent their disjointed social lives. Over a drink, they relived the day. Nothing seemed quite as terrible now that it was over. The television crew could describe how Charlie had peeled back Aaron's scalp, lifted the plate from his skull and sat it down like an ashtray. Everyone talked about the hours of tension when they could barely breathe.

Charlie rode home on his motorbike, through the cold, empty streets, ready to party. Luckily, the next day, Friday, was his day off. He couldn't have slept, even though his neck and shoulders and every joint and muscle down to his legs and feet ached with tiredness. He never needed more than six hours' sleep. If nothing else was happening, he would stay up and watch television or write reports and correspondence. That night, his house was still rocking with Peter Nakaji's farewell bash.

Nakaji wasn't surprised to see Charlie become the life of the party after a tough day. On his second night in Sydney, Charlie had told him they had to go to a farewell celebration for a nurse who was leaving the hospital. After operating all day, they went home for dinner and Charlie fell asleep. Nakaji thought the night was over but after twenty minutes, Charlie jumped up, pushed on his glasses and said, 'Let's go.' They danced until four in the morning. Another night they operated until 4 am then went to the Bourbon & Beefsteak in Kings Cross for a plate of garlic prawns. Next day at the hospital no one would come near them but Charlie was clear-headed and energetic. Nakaji wondered if he could keep up the pace for six months.

Yes, Charlie was controversial. He didn't have great insight into his own personality and he sometimes blundered about, but to Nakaji that was endearing. 'If I needed to cross a minefield, I'd take Charlie Teo with me and push him ahead because I know he'd set off all the mines.'

Now Nakaji was leaving Sydney convinced that Charlie was the most talented neurosurgeon in the country when it came to removing brain tumours. He had worked with him on so many cases that he was willing to stick his neck out. Charlie reminded him of the American neurosurgeon Gazi Yasargil in many ways. With patients he was honest but always hopeful. In surgery he had endurance and a perfect sense of timing, a willingness to persist gently for as long as necessary. His minimally invasive techniques were impressive and his results were the best Nakaji had seen.

Recalling that day's operation, Nakaji said, 'It was the reverse of building a ship in a bottle: he had to dismantle it inside. The tumour was very sticky. There are a lot of tracks connecting the two sides of the brain, and Charlie had to find a route down to the tumour and a way to get it out bit by bit.'

As the tumour bled and Aaron's brain swelled, he said, 'I could tell Charlie was more nervous, more alert and hyped up during that operation than I'd seen him. It wasn't five minutes of trouble, it was hours and hours, like slogging through a storm.

'It was like a storm coming in and then clearing. It got harder to see as the clouds and rain closed in, and then he kept working on the tumour until the clouds began to break. You could feel the tenor of the room change. We could have decided to back out and stop the bleeding and come back another day. But the second time is not as good as the first and you risk leaving a big blood clot.'

Nakaji had heard Aaron play the piano before his operation and he'd said to Charlie, 'Not to worry you or anything, but I think he's a really good pianist.' He knew that would put pressure on Charlie. 'He tries to tailor his work to the patient, not to the disease. He remembers people by their personal details. In some respects, he is more like an American surgeon – but I don't see patients come out laughing as they do with him. By the end of a consultation, people look as though they've decided to buy a holiday home.'

As far as Nakaji could see, Charlie had only one flaw: 'That incessant John Denver music. I used to like John Denver before I knew Charlie.'

17

VISITATIONS

The first person Aaron saw when he opened his eyes was Brian, a solid, monk-like figure meditating with his eyes closed beside the bed. Even then, he sensed the sweet irony. Waking up in a new phase of being alive and there was his father, whom he had never called 'Father'.

Brian had wanted to be there when Aaron woke up properly. While the others recovered at the pub, he sat still and silent in a chair and waited. The first words he heard Aaron speak were, 'I'm bored.' Brian could see that after all his son had endured, his mind was working inside his battered body. He asked a nurse how long he would be in intensive care. Even through the fog, Aaron could hear her say they'd keep him for as short a time as possible because that's where the worst germs were.

'What next?' he wondered.

When Gail returned from the pub at three in the morning, Brian offered to drive her home, and she, finally spent, allowed him to. Little willy-willies of dust blew in the streets and they were both pleased not to be alone. Before dawn, Brian left Gail and her car at her parents' house, caught a train to the city and a bus to Randwick, and trudged back to Aaron's bedside, where he dozed in the chair.

Just as he had felt no fear going into surgery, Aaron was not amazed or elated to find he was alive. Gail's pre-operation warning to ignore the white light that drew people towards death seemed to have been unnecessary; he could remember nothing since being sedated. All he wanted was ice to soothe his dry, ulcerated mouth and throat. A nurse slid water and ice slivers between his lips, and then he was able to concentrate on how disjointed the rest of his body seemed.

A nurse came every hour to shine a light in his eyes, make sure his pupils responded, check that he knew who and where he was and that everything still moved. Every time he drifted towards sleep, he fell into violent nightmares, an abstract inferno of horrors, and woke frightened and dripping with sweat. The tubes holding him to the bed would loosen, summoning the nurse with their beeps.

Brian was by no means the oddest figure he would see in the coming hours and days. His swollen brain developed a double life, swinging between reality and a carnival of hallucinations even when he was awake. David Wansbrough appeared sitting at a piano, throwing his hands up and down in an exaggerated honky-tonk style of play, grinning and laughing. The real David couldn't play the piano but had inspired so much of Aaron's musical composition. Suddenly, David made way for Peter Crisp, who had been Aaron's minder, driver and crowd controller through his month of illness. Standing with his back to Aaron, Peter seemed to be mixing something on a table and

Aaron wondered if he was making a jelly. Then Peter spun around as though on a turntable and tipped a bowl towards Aaron, showering him with fiery, sparkling dust.

At the same moment, Aaron broke out in a real sweat again. This time, a wave of warmth and calm swept through him, and he felt all the disconnections in his body being healed. Perhaps there was a practical explanation for his sensations. The nurse who admitted him to intensive care at 5.30 am on 17 August noted that he was hypothermic, shivering and hypertensive, and that he required 'active heating', which probably meant covering him with heated blankets. But Aaron preferred to interpret the sensation as the most potent of all the spiritual healing gifts he had received. During the long, uncertain hours of surgery, Peter had asked the universal powers he believed in to show him some tangible way of helping. And now it seemed as if he had assisted the surgeon with his magical potion.

Aaron started to re-enter reality in the high-dependency unit when one of the nurses gave him a bed bath and brought him toast and tea at one o'clock on Saturday morning. It was a thrill to eat. Propped up in bed, he felt as if his head were a great weight that could topple off his shoulders. Trying to sleep again, he kept starting awake and watching the clock: 3.08 . . . 3.09 . . . 3.15 . . . 3.30.

Among the CDs by his bed was a collection of Beethoven's last five piano sonatas, written when the composer was at the height of his powers. Aaron abandoned sleep, put on the expensive headphones his friends Steve and Andi had lent him, and listened to every movement. Four hours of music helped to clear his brain and carried him through to morning.

Within a few hours, he was sitting up and detached from most of his monitors. 'Dr Teo said you could go home today,' said a nurse, and when Aaron laughed, she added, 'No, really, he did.'

Aaron hadn't even contemplated standing up when, a short time later, in walked Charlie with his four daughters. He had taken the girls with him on rounds since they were babies because he wanted them to be comfortable with his work and they brought life into the wards.

'G'day, old son. You're looking good,' he said. He turned to chat to the nurses, then spoke to Aaron again. 'We were going to send you home today. Have you been for a walk?'

'I didn't know I could. I'll give it a go,' Aaron said.

An idea formed as he spoke. He swung his legs out of the bed while a nurse was still detaching him from the drips. His head wasn't bandaged and wasn't all that painful but his stitches and blood-encrusted hair made him feel fragile. At first he wondered if he could make it to the door. Once he was standing and his legs began working, he was more confident.

'Bugger it. Let's give it a go,' he thought.

He stepped carefully along the corridor in his shorts, T-shirt and socks, with Charlie and his nurse Kate at his side. Gail and Amy followed. People appeared out of doorways to watch and follow and cheer him on. He tried not to think about how far he was from his bed.

'You should see my piano,' he said casually. 'I've got a piano down here and I could play it for you.'

Charlie knew about the piano but he hadn't seen the great pianist perform. When they reached the piano room, at the far end of the floor from the high-dependency ward, a small crowd had gathered. Without much thought, Aaron began. Scarlatti's Sonata in C, from the early seventeenth century, was one of the flashiest pieces he had learned for his album. Fast, bright and spirit-lifting, it tested his dexterity but it was also short. He had no doubt he could play. His fingers had been running along an imaginary keyboard in bed and he could feel the music flowing back into them.

He moved into a second piece he had recorded just before he fell ill. Chopin's well-known Waltz No. 7 in C sharp minor was romantic with a tinge of sadness. He knew his audience must see this as a huge challenge for him, but it was so easy. He was energised, his head felt empty and his mind sharp.

Charlie stood entranced. He had been relieved to see Aaron wiggle his fingers and toes when he woke up from the operation, but he expected to see some damage the next day. Aaron was as pale as a ghost and day two was when patients had maximum swelling after an operation, so if he were going to do badly, it would be today or tomorrow. People could say they felt normal but when it got down to the nitty-gritty of doing something complex, that's when you saw subtle deficits. Aaron might look good, feel good and move his fingers dexterously, but it was only thirty-six hours since Charlie had been elbow-deep in his blood. Now he was watching a concert performance. His disbelief was so strong that at first he thought Aaron had prerecorded the music and was playing it back. Only when he stopped mid-phrase and started again was Charlie convinced.

Erica Jacobsen, the registrar on the ward, stood by the piano as Aaron played again later that day. She was astonished. He had played beautifully before but now each note was enunciated and the music rang with especial clarity. Charlie deserved enormous credit, she thought, because he was always so gentle. Any neurosurgeon could have done the operation – *she* could have done the operation – but few could have achieved such a remarkable result.

Aaron felt the same way. There was such freedom in his head. His mind seemed to open up, his memory was crystal clear, and he could play seemingly anything. He was almost embarrassed by how healthy he felt, as though he should be a bit more messed up and melancholic. But he couldn't pretend.

Aaron didn't go home that day. He was still weak and needed observation. His bed was beside the window and, as the first light appeared next morning, he looked at the city skyline and thought, 'I want to get back out there, that crazy town, and conquer it and get on with things.'

Full of lightness and hope, he put on his headphones to listen to Bach's violin concertos. He always found Bach warming. Just a few minutes into the Violin Concerto in A Minor, he realised he was hearing in a new way. The music flooded through him to his core. He could hear every thread of texture with clarity, from the top of the violins to the bottom of the bass. It wasn't volume; the sound was brighter and more alive. He had a sudden grasp of what he'd been through, fear giving way to joy, mixed with sadness to discover that he had been plugging away with only just enough hearing to be a musician. Sobs jolted out of him.

A few visitors came to see Aaron but, now the high drama was over, people seemed to have let go, gone back to their own lives. The camera crew was gone, too. Gail had to return to her family and work in Brisbane, but until then she sat by Aaron's bed. Walking with her son, she noticed how much taller he seemed than before his operation, as if a weight had lifted and allowed him to stand up straight again. Marjorie, his grandmother, looked at him with a warm, weathered smile, as if he had emerged from a war zone.

When Elliot Bullock arrived, Aaron was lying on his back ready to give a pep talk.

'My little angel,' he said. 'I did it. You knew I would. There's no stopping us, is there?'

Elliot sat on the bed while they listened to the cricket Test on the radio and talked about his training: the drills he should do, the overs he should be bowling. Aaron seemed so unchanged that it was easy to carry on as usual. A counsellor who had promised to see him in case he was traumatised by surgery popped her head in and left, clearly unneeded.

A dignified white-haired man arrived, looking to Aaron like some sort of prophet. He was Erwin Berney, a Hungarian-born teacher who had helped to bring anthroposophy to Australia after the Nazis tramped through Europe, and used his scientific training to start the famous non-profit biodynamic Demeter Bakery in Sydney. Aaron knew him as an elder of Glenaeon School, a friend of his mother and a supporter of his music.

Fearful that he would find Aaron bandaged and semi-conscious, instead Erwin saw him talking on the phone, like someone who did not belong in hospital.

'Aaron, this is fantastic!' he said. He had come to tell him how important his survival was. Rudolf Steiner taught that, beginning in 1879, this was the age of the Archangel Saint Michael, a medieval knight, dragon slayer and ambassador of Christ. Aaron had always helped others, with his music and his generosity. Having come back from the precipice of a life-threatening challenge, slaying his own dragon, he was now an active helper of Saint Michael and had a duty to work for the benefit of the world.

Erwin's statement confirmed Aaron's feelings of destiny and Aaron wanted to say something glorious in return. He put the headphones over Erwin's ears and played him the Bach violin concerto that had been so profound a few hours earlier. The older man enjoyed the music but couldn't comprehend its importance in the same way.

Aaron's friend Simon Creedy insisted on driving him to Coogee beach for an ice-cream the following day. Aaron tried to stop his head from bouncing as the car spun round the bends. They bought their cones and walked down to the concrete promenade above the sand, where a few people were strolling and seagulls were wheeling in the cold breeze. An ordinary day at the beach, but not for Aaron. He might as well have been on a different planet. A week earlier, the scene, with its sand and sea and distant horizon, had looked like a flat, pale painting on a wall. Now everything was rendered as if in super-3D. The depth of field had opened up and the colour was rich. It was almost too intense, and he felt as if he were a child seeing everything for the first time with brand-new eyes, unclouded by familiarity and the distractions of life.

'Is this what you always see?' he asked Simon. 'You lucky bastard.'

Simon laughed. He was a graphic designer and one of Aaron's most visually sensitive friends, but all he saw was a normal day, chilly and overcast.

Much as he wanted to, Aaron couldn't expect other people to share his wonder. Just as he had faced the possibility of death on his own, he had to return to life, step by step, on his own. But he was not quite alone. The little blonde girl who had appeared to him at his apartment came back. Instead of beseeching him with her hands raised, this time she was dancing and laughing. She seemed to be checking on him, celebrating his recovery and bringing more visitors.

A parade of other figures flowed past most of the time Aaron was awake. They inhabited the blank area in his left field of vision, like a television screen. Giant doctors in white coats and size twenty-eight shoes went by, so tall that he couldn't see their faces until they bent down to peer in at him. Nurses and school-children crowded past. Then there was the cowboy. Dressed like a Hollywood hero – perhaps John Wayne – in baggy trousers, boots, spurs, pistols and a hat, he came and went like the others, looking in through the 'window' without trying to interact. Then he turned up when Aaron was making a cup of tea in the kitchen on his ward. Mostly, Aaron watched the apparitions with a vague curiosity, but after a while he grew tired of their constant in-trusion. For the first time, he spoke out loud.

'Are you going to kill me?'

The cowboy didn't answer but pulled his gun out of its holster and pointed it at Aaron's head. Then, with a wide grin, he dropped it slowly to his side. If he represented Aaron's sub-conscious, he was clearly a symbol of reprieve.

At night, the images changed. The window was on the left-hand side of his bed and, as his peripheral vision took in the quietened streets of Randwick, he saw a much more exotic scene. He could have been in a Russian city. A red-brick apartment building was transformed into the city gates; its roof, a gold-encrusted castle wall. A branch hanging over a garbage bin became a guard and the street lights washed everything in a magical glow.

Aaron tried not to question the people and places he was seeing but they prompted some deep thoughts. Everyone has had the experience of having a car horn or an unexplained bang fit into a dream, clattering plates in the kitchen sink turning into a car crash in their narrative. Most people don't think any more of it, but to Aaron's heightened awareness, those coincidences were signs of another dimension just out of sight of our daily lives.

How else could we pre-empt those about-to-happen sounds and make them fit into our dreams? Where else did these strangers and distant scenes appear from? Of course, they only appeared in the window in his peripheral vision caused by his tumour.

With his eyes closed, his brain set off another, more abstract pattern. He saw a rolling sphere covered with a grid of symmetrical green blocks, some short, some tall, which seemed to extend infinitely in all directions. It was so clear and precise that he could draw it, like a city of miniature towers. He learned from his stepfather that a computer motherboard looked just like that, with endless X and Y grids of clustered blocks where the information is stored. It was like watching the neurons in his brain reconnect and start to send clear messages again. No wonder he couldn't sleep.

'Oh, people have hallucinations from the dex,' said Erica Jacobsen when Aaron told her about his 'visitors'. She heard stories about odd visions all the time, some of them violent and frightening. She had even had some herself as a trainee, when she had worked for three days without sleep and started seeing animal faces in a patient's brain during surgery. The neurosurgeon she was assisting told her to stay awake by sewing closed the scalp.

Aaron's hallucinations had a different origin.

'When you lose vision and you don't know that you've lost it, often your brain will insert things for you,' Jacobsen told me. 'Aaron would see quite bizarre people in his peripheral vision after the operation. It takes a while for it all to heal but it's also pushing on areas of your brain which don't just deal with how you see but how all that information gets formed into images in your brain. There's this huge area next to your visual cortex called the association cortex that processes all those messages, and that's where a lot of hallucinations come in. You're missing a connection, so the connection's coming from somewhere else and it misinforms [you on] what's going on. It's one of those areas of neurophysiology that ten years ago in the textbooks there was virtually nothing on and then, between editions, suddenly there's an explosion of information. We still don't really understand it.'

Aaron understood the medical explanation for the phenomenon he was experiencing but he believed he had been given a glimpse of a world that was usually behind a curtain. Even when he looked back, with no drugs in his brain, he held on to his theory. Although his stories sometimes sounded like scenes from a science fiction movie, he was making his usual effort to decipher meaning rather than nothingness behind the sets where we play our daily life.

'The way these things presented themselves to me, there was this incredible sense that they were there all the time,' he said. 'I really felt they were peeking in, having a look, being happy, dancing around, pointing the gun at me, just as a distraction from what they normally do. It came across to me as though this was a dimension that we don't see and these things are ever present and guiding us. I didn't have a feeling that they were my own creation, that they were constructed for me. It wasn't a product of my mind. It felt like the place from which I've come, to which I'm going back, and there was something more real about it than this crazy ride I was on.'

18

ANATOMY OF A MIRACLE

'How's it feeling?' Charlie was behind his desk with a grin on his face and a jar of chocolate M&Ms at his side. He had glanced at his neat needlework on the back of Aaron's head, from where the stitches had just been removed. 'It's great that things have gone so well. I bet your family's really happy. I'm pretty certain we got all the tumour out and we'll give you an MRI soon to make sure. I want you to start exercising and get back into it.'

Aaron reminded Charlie of his warning that he wouldn't be the same person after the operation. But he was playing the piano and his peripheral vision seemed to be returning. Everything else was working. Charlie described the crisis in the theatre and the solutions he had tried without success. Aaron pictured, with difficulty, his head cut open, his flooding brain, his obliviousness to the intimate struggle inside his body.

'So, what on earth happened?'

'Aaron . . .' Charlie paused. 'I have no idea.'

Aaron would always remember that answer. It seemed that at some point his brain had just decided to turn around. Charlie was the champion, with his skill and care and determination, but perhaps there was something else: Aaron's own determination, the prayers said for him, his conversations with a greater power that decided he was worth keeping. Charlie was happy to agree. There were good outcomes he couldn't fully explain and Aaron's was one of them. Yes, call it a miracle.

Brian had borrowed a van again to take Aaron and his piano home. They left with a reminder from Charlie that Aaron should take his dexamethasone. Nothing was said about the five-thousand-dollar fee that Charlie had mentioned when they first met. Nothing would ever be said. Charlie treated the case as a public emergency and didn't charge the cash-strapped pianist a cent.

Back at his apartment in the city, Aaron had the strange sensation of walking into his old life as a transformed person. Opening his front door, he found that his neighbours Steve and Andi had vacuumed and filled the emptiness with a table and cane chairs they had dug out of the building's storeroom. Visitors would need somewhere to sit, they reasoned.

Aaron was still not to be left alone, in case he suffered a seizure, so Peter Crisp arrived with his rucksack and rolled out his sleeping bag on the living-room floor. Every few hours that first night he called out, 'Aaron.' But they were both desperately weary and, at last, Aaron slept through the night. In a dream, he saw his mother and sister playing games in an unfamiliar house on a hill. He woke refreshed and rang Gail to share his contentment.

His hallucinations didn't follow him home but life kept

surprising him. Sitting at his desk, where he had first got word of the tumour, looking down the hall where the little blonde girl used to make her appearances, he realised everything was different. Where there had been a blur, he saw a long corridor with a door at the end. The dimensions and lines and colours were sharply defined.

His desk had planes and angles he hadn't noticed. A bowl of fruit on his desk was even more striking. The oranges and apples were so vivid and beautiful. Aaron devised tests for whether Peter was seeing things in the same way. Is the red part of an apple brighter than the yellow? Is this blue darker than that? He set all kinds of parameters of contrast and shade. In the end, he had to concede that Peter saw everything he saw but couldn't appreciate its richness. Sometimes Aaron's head spun with the intensity and he had to close his eyes.

Normality bored him. Other people's conversations were banal. Daily life seemed trivial. He felt like an astronaut who had looked down from a great height and seen the silliness of men's affairs. As usual, he had plans. Most of all, he told everyone, he wanted to live unselfishly. It was a pure, if not altogether realistic, intention.

Even while he was in hospital, he had decided to stage a comeback concert in Sydney to thank all his friends and family for their support and show how well he was. Peter was organising an annual country ball at his home near the town of Yass three weeks later – the Canberra Youth Orchestra would be playing, so why not join them? Aaron was reluctant at first to travel hundreds of kilometres into the bush and ask his friends to follow, but Peter had been so kind it was hard to say no. It was a great chance to be a musician again.

On Saturday 15 September 2001, Aaron caught the train to

Yass. The concert was being held in the corrugated-iron hall that Peter had built for big events, and it filled with locals who went to the ball every year and a heartwarming number of people who had come from Sydney and further afield to see Aaron. Peter, the dinner-suited master of ceremonies, told the audience, 'Tonight is a celebration. Only four weeks ago Aaron McMillan was diagnosed with a brain tumour that was one of the largest, most complicated brain tumours known in medical history. Tonight, we actually see a miracle. Very fortunately, Aaron has come through his surgery unscathed. Tonight he's performing Mozart's Piano Concerto in C, Number 21.'

Only the tiny arc of bare skin amid his hair reminded them how recently he had been at risk. The crew from *Australian Story* arrived to film a happy ending before putting the story to air. They managed to capture the one mistake he made all night, but Aaron didn't care – his heart was light and his brain was full of music. One cloud hung over the evening. On 11 September, two American jets had been hijacked by Arab terrorists and flown into the World Trade Center towers in New York. Others had crashed into the Pentagon in Washington and into a field in Pennsylvania. Aaron thought about the hours it had taken Charlie to save his life and the instant mass deaths caused by one violent act. It was an equation with no balance. But twelve days after his performance, almost a million people took inspiration from his appearance on *Australian Story*.

The pathology tests on Aaron's tumour had already confirmed that it was a hemangiopericytoma, the rare and idiosyncratic variety that grew from the membrane around the brain rather than the brain tissue itself but could not truthfully be described as benign. Charlie had made it clear to Aaron that there was a chance – a small chance – that it could recur. Aaron was anxious that his first MRI after leaving hospital would show that some of the murky white cloud had been left behind. Handed the envelope at the hospital, he couldn't bear to wait until his appointment with Charlie the next day so he hurried to the window, pulled out the scans and held them against the fading light. Right where the tumour had been, he could see a little ball of white. His stomach went into a spasm of fear.

Next morning, Charlie took the scans and held them up with one hand while he talked on the phone and scooped M&Ms from the jar. He seemed to take forever, turning the images and peering at microscopic spots.

'I've got one word for you, Aaron,' he said at last. 'Celebrate. It looks fantastic.'

Aaron started to breathe again. The white patch was the tip of a bone that came up into the head, Charlie explained. Completely normal and nothing to worry about. Aaron was still in shock.

'Well, what do I do now?'

'Come kayaking with me.'

A few weeks later, in the spring-warmed air, Charlie and Aaron took to Sydney Harbour. Charlie liked to show his patients they were capable of strenuous exercise, and Aaron didn't need coddling. They argued about who was stronger and who paddled harder. Charlie put Aaron in the front seat and sat back in an exaggerated pose of relaxation while his patient pulled the boat around Shark Island. They went out often as Aaron grew fitter and they came to know each other as equals. Charlie began to perceive Aaron as an exceptional young man with a highly developed social conscience as well as a healthy ego. Charlie might work his butt off to save people's lives, but he also remembered himself as an average, self-centred 24-year-old wrapped up in his career, girls and motorbikes. Aaron seemed to have another, more ethereal dimension.

Aaron loved those mornings, with cold water flying in his face and dolphins looping along beside them. He enjoyed showing off his youthful strength against Charlie's muscled and trained expertise. But he felt vulnerable. He was tired and he heard tiny gurgles and squirts in the empty spaces inside his head.

Turning around in the boat one morning, he looked at Charlie. 'I could still die from this, couldn't I?'

'I'm not going to let you die,' said Charlie.

For Aaron and those close to him, the risk that his cancer could recur was of minuscule importance compared with his return to wholeness. Everyone felt they had played a part in his salvation and Aaron was pleased to share the triumph. Friends were elated, as if they had stepped off the earth, as if lightning had struck, as if they all had a second chance at life.

Aaron was no longer an invalid but relatives and friends still felt responsible for guiding his recovery and his future. Brian arranged a meeting at Aaron's apartment with his grandfather, Frank Robinson, and his friends Stuart Gentle, David Wansbrough and Peter Crisp. They discussed a plan for him to teach music, pay off his swelling debts, buy a house and become 'normal'. Though they meant well, Aaron was furious, and resented Brian's attempt to play the unearned role of father.

Gail interpreted the tumour as a sign that Aaron had to get back to basics and focus on what was most important to him. She sensed a change in him: 'I think he feels now that time is finite and that if he wants to get these big things done, he has to set about doing it with renewed vigour and perception and priorities.' Andi also noticed that Aaron's values had changed, that his thinking seemed more global, that he felt a duty to use his 'bonus time' to help the world. He hoped Aaron would not become a slave to his sense of purpose.

Aaron thought endlessly about the meaning of his near-death but it didn't feel like a burden. It was just as Erwin Berney had said: with his second life he could do anything, be anything, if he believed in it strongly enough. The only way to return all the love he had received was by dedicating himself to other people. Six thousand letters and emails arrived in the months after his television appearance. Charlie would see two hundred patients as a result of the show. Already, Aaron felt he had helped.

Undeterred by the realists, he held to the vision he'd had in his hospital bed. He would compose, and change the whole conception of Western music. Yet he cared too much about interaction with people to give up his other ambitions. He would be a mentor to musicians and a communicator through music. He would make it all into a profitable business.

First, he had to go back into the ABC studio with Yossi Gabbay and put together the CD he had abandoned a few weeks earlier. They worked quickly but carefully. On 22 July 2002, Aaron launched his double CD, *Time Within*, at the Eugene Goossens Hall, where he had recorded the music. His liner notes read:

As I began to record the works I realised the importance of allowing time in the music, being very conscious of silences and pauses between the notes. I wanted to find a balance between playing the music and breathing some space into the music . . . My friend David Wansbrough suggests 'a continuum of music where we approach the silence of the future'.

It was a year since he had left this room in distress, returning a few weeks later with the ABC crew to play Rachmaninov, perhaps for the last time. Now he gazed ahead and the future looked vast.

19

ENCORE

When Aaron was twelve, his mother and stepfather took him to the Sydney Opera House for a concert by Dimitris Sgouros, a dazzling young Greek pianist. From his seat, the piano lid obscured Aaron's view of Sgouros, but he was so elated by the nineteen-year-old virtuoso's performance that he left believing he, too, could scale the highest musical peaks. He pictured himself on the Opera House stage one day.

As he grew older, reason argued that it wasn't so easy. The Opera House had its annual seasons for the Sydney Symphony Orchestra, Musica Viva and the Australian Chamber Orchestra. The ABC held its piano series there, mostly bringing in international artists; local solo pianists had to rely on promoters and the opportunities were thin.

Aaron's unconventional route into music had not endeared him to the establishment. He had never been interested in sitting in a studio rehearsing to an infinite degree of perfection and following a schedule dictated by a manager. He had seen too many young pianists end up doing the rounds of clubs and bars, or dropping out of music altogether because of the stress of competition and an inability to create their own opportunities. He might not be the best pianist of his generation, but unless he was playing for an audience he couldn't see much point in playing. Music was communication. So, he began by considering where he wanted to play and for whom, and then he set about making it happen.

By the time he decided to present himself at the Opera House, the only Australian pianists to have given solo recitals in the Concert Hall were the world-famous Roger Woodward and the eccentric David Helfgott, after the film *Shine* had made him a figure of popular culture. Aaron was undeterred. Rather than wait for a promoter to issue an invitation, he booked the hall. It was most unusual for a musician to organise his own event on this ambitious a scale. Community groups often hired the hall for concerts, and individuals sometimes brought in a small private audience, but a full-scale concert? There were a few tut-tuts from the conservatives in the music world but others agreed that young musicians had to create opportunities for themselves and they cheered Aaron's gutsiness. He used his mailing list to contact as many people as possible who had seen him perform, bought a recording, written to him after *Australian Story* or known him as a friend. Never before had his potential audience been so large.

Over several months, Aaron sold more than a thousand of the Concert Hall's twenty-six hundred seats and the Opera House box office sold several hundred more. To cover the massive production costs, he used all the money he could make from selling CDs and pre-selling live CDs of the Opera House concert, as well as money from private patrons who sponsored his recordings or simply wrote a cheque because they believed in him, without much expectation of any financial return. He whittled a program out of music chosen by friends. Most pieces were favourites by Schubert and Chopin and Brahms and Liszt, with a few surprises that held special meaning for him and his intimates.

As he began to practise, he learned that the Opera House had just taken delivery of a new nine-foot Steinway grand piano from Hamburg. Before it would be ready for the public, it needed to be played for eighty hours. Julie Seaton, the Opera House events manager, was about to ring the Sydney Conservatorium to invite some students in when she remembered that Aaron would be the first to perform on it. Would he like to break it in?

With a twenty-four-hour pass, he was able to slip into the deserted Opera House and down through the wood-panelled corridors of rehearsal rooms to the conductor's room. The glossy black piano stood in the middle of the room, its keys untouched until Aaron's hands made them resonate with Liszt, Chopin and Schubert. Looking through the strip of narrow windows at the Harbour Bridge, he saw how extravagant his Opera House dream had been, and felt proud that it was about to come true as his twenty-sixth birthday slid by.

A few times in those months, he caught a train to the wide suburban street where Neta Maughan was teaching yet another generation of young pianists. Miss Maughan, as he usually called her, had become a friend and coach and reliable critic. Late one night, he crouched over the piano in her music room, among the armchairs and piles of sheet music, while she sat back and listened silently as he played through his program. Every now and then, she interrupted and made him repeat a passage with different pedalling or more emphasis or more slowly.

'You have to think of the acoustics in that huge hall and give the audience's ears time to catch up,' she said.

From the day Aaron had walked into her house ten years earlier, she had remarked on his great facility for the instrument but often had wanted more colour in his expression. Now, with the tumour removed from his brain, she knew why. She could already hear more range in his tone. His plan for the Opera House was wildly ambitious, as always, but she wouldn't try to dissuade him. Rather, she would be there, breathing every note, savouring his achievement.

A week before the concert, dragging himself home at 2 am after hours of practice, Aaron knew he hadn't mastered every stroke and nuance of his music. He should have practised for a year and memorised the music three months earlier. But he comforted himself with the knowledge that most musicians cut corners. With more than five hundred performances racked up, he knew he would give the audience everything he had.

On Monday 25 February 2003, seventeen months after the operation and two weeks after his twenty-sixth birthday, Aaron walked onto the stage. In a carefully fitted charcoal-grey suit and long-sleeved white T-shirt, rather than the traditional bow tie and tails, he cut an elegant but unassuming figure. There had been no dress rehearsal, so this was the first time he had stood here and looked into the steep auditorium. He gave the audience a light bow and a smile before sitting down; eighteen hundred fans replied with an emotional rush of applause. He could have peered into any row and seen people whose throats were tight with pride and disbelief: his mother, his father, his brother and sister, his grandparents, his surgeon, dozens of friends, hundreds of acquaintances and strangers. Some were seeing their first live classical concert.

Aaron had trained himself long before against stage fright. Whenever someone asked if he got nervous, he said firmly, 'No, never.' If he had said, 'Oh, sometimes,' it would have left the door open to doubt. If he'd said, 'Always,' what could he expect? Perhaps it was the same trick that had guided his reactions to his illness and so disconcerted Charlie.

He began the concert delicately with Schubert's Impromptu in F minor, written the year before the composer died at thirty-one from syphilis, a period when he wrote some of his finest works. Aaron knew he looked relaxed, even detached, at the piano. There was no flamboyance to his movements. But, through his fingertips, he was intent on giving his audience the first thrill that would carry them with him. He then moved into two compositions by Chopin and a passionate Rachmaninov Prelude in G minor.

'So far, pretty good,' he thought. The next piece was very important to him. Intermezzo in A by Brahms was the music Neta Maughan wanted played at her funeral, and was her favourite piano composition. They had been through it together many times but suddenly Aaron had a complete memory lapse. At a tricky point, where one chord changed in the repetition of a passage and led down another path, he made the change too soon. Of all the times and places! Still, he was a master of cover-ups and only a few people, including Neta, would notice. He berated himself during interval in his dressing room. Back onstage, he moved ahead smoothly.

The exuberant second half of the concert began with the most physically demanding piece, the *Spanish Rhapsody* by Liszt, which he had been playing since he was seventeen. Its exhibitionism called for enormous energy. Sweat flew from his face, catching the light, as the piece's last minutes built to their dramatic ending. He stood to roars from the audience and staggered into a bow, reaching out for the piano in an exaggerated gesture that he hoped was comical. People close enough could see the exertion on his pale, wet forehead. It was a relief when he sat and touched the keys.

Towards the end of the night, the music took a more personal turn. Aaron was joined onstage by Sylvie Renaud-Calmel, a French-born soprano and close friend. She turned the pages as he played a piece by her late father, Roger Calmel. The program finale was *Evryali*, the Xenakis composition Aaron had recorded into his piano the morning before his operation. He lost his way in the rapid, pounding chords that took his hands all over the keyboard at once. But he knew that few pianists got through the storm of notes without some improvisation and, when he rose, the applause was just as wild as the music had been.

Still the concert wasn't over. The encore was for himself, though some in the audience would recognise it as the theme from *Australian Story* and others would simply enjoy its calming romanticism after the madness of Xenakis. Rachmaninov's Prelude in D, the music Aaron had played in hospital until he knew every note, not sure if he would ever play again, could now be shared. How could he finish any other way?

The last notes, soft and optimistic, hung in the auditorium until they were overtaken by a loud rain of clapping, hooting and whistles. The audience leaped to their feet as Aaron's teenage sister came out to give him an extravagant bouquet of flowers.

'Thank Christ it's over,' he thought. Fatigue obliterated elation and he could only hope Amy was enjoying her moment in the spotlight.

In the faded green room, he was polite but dazed as his guests fussed around him. He knew he'd given them pleasure and that was enough. Gail was torn between wanting to whisk her son home to bed and savouring his performance at a concert for which she had provided neither money nor food, as she had at earlier events. Marjorie and Frank simply smiled on their grandson. Brian stood back as usual.

Out of his element, Charlie still felt like a philistine, but watching Aaron play with the precision and speed of an athlete had filled him with admiration. One thought throbbed in his head all night: 'Thank God I didn't cut into his brain.'

20

PILGRIMS

'I can feel this guy's pain,' said Charlie. It was ten o'clock on a March morning in 2003, and he was looking into the mess that an operation three months earlier had left in the brain of a New Zealander in his forties named Michael Bartrom. But Charlie was talking about the surgeon's pain and the panic he must have felt when he began to lose control. 'He hit the carotid artery. There's blood everywhere, he's got clips all over the place as he tried to stop it.' Most neurosurgeons have made a devastating micro-slip like that. Charlie is no exception – 'but probably not for ten years. Fortunately, you tend to do it earlier in your career than later. I'd rather leave some tumour than hit the carotid.'

He pushed through the shiny white brain tissue, matted with grey scar tissue from the previous operation, and came eventually to a distinct, pale, plum-sized tumour. He eased the bipolar around its surface and sang along with Simon and Garfunkel. An orchestra of air-conditioning, sucking and beeping sounds almost drowned out his masked performance.

'Great song!' Charlie yelled over the last words of 'America'.

His nurse, Kate, rolled in trays of instruments, set up the micro-scope, opened packets of swabs and came back with the staff lunch menu. She went through the options: steak, sandwiches, spinach and ricotta in filo pastry.

'Why don't we get some Chinese take-out?' shouted Charlie without raising his eyes from the lens. Orders placed, Kate went to pathology with a chunk of tumour floating lifelessly in saline. At 12.20 pm, Charlie stretched his shoulders and said, 'Finished. I've got all the tumour.'

Another hour would pass while he roughly sewed the dura mater over the open brain, replaced a large square of skull with the old-fashioned screws used by the previous surgeon and closed the S-shaped incision in the scalp with neat stitches. The man's head looked like a soccer ball. The anaesthetist, Peter Isert, had already begun shutting off the flow of drugs and the patient began to twitch as the clamp came off his temples.

'He will wake up immediately,' said Charlie. 'Other anaes-thetists can do that but Peter can get them to wake up and ask for a cup of tea.'

A solid man with crinkly hair and glasses, Isert gave the impression of being laidback as he whispered on his mobile phone while his equipment suspended patients between life and death. He had begun training as a surgeon until one day when he assisted on a haemorrhoidectomy. The patient lay with his legs in stirrups and as the surgeon tied off the bulging veins, he said, 'Look at those, Pete. Aren't they beauties?' Isert realised he could never find haemorrhoids interesting. He looked across at the anaesthetist, watching the monitor with his feet up on the life-sustaining machinery, and knew what he wanted to do.

'Living physiology,' he called it – studying the individual quirks of a patient's blood pressure and respiration. He was one of two anaesthetists who took it in turns to work on Charlie's private cases. They didn't need to talk much during operations and if Charlie's music was too loud, Isert simply turned up the volume on his machine. He saw his ability to control conscious-ness as a privilege, an art and a mystery. Giving patients a crisp, comfortable awakening within five or ten minutes of the opera-tion's completion also allowed the neurosurgeon to see quickly how well the brain was working. Could they move, speak, control their eyes?

'Charlie's patients certainly look good,' he said, 'because their incisions tend to be small and the minimally invasive approach means minimal damage to other tissue. The same as a smart bomb: there's less collateral damage. When you drop a bomb, you don't want to kill two million people. It's more a philosophy than a method.'

By the time that particular morning's patient woke up, Charlie was in the staffroom, hurrying through a plastic tub of com-bination chow mein, smearing each mouthful with chilli sauce and grunting with pleasure. For five minutes, he leaned his blue-capped head against the wall and slept. Compared with his old schoolmate Trevor Danos, who had gone into law, with its harbour views and corporate lunches, Charlie had taken the unglamorous option. He didn't think about it that way. Eyes suddenly open, he looked at the time, just after two, and went to scrub his hands and forearms before re-entering the dim, cold theatre for the next operation.

Thanks to the media coverage of the past few years and his

success with Aaron McMillan, Charlie was busier than ever and seeing more people for whom he was the last hope. He sat up into the night scrutinising their scans, spent more hours on the phone listening to their stories and telling most of them why he couldn't help. The heartache was worth it, for the one in ten he could offer some future.

His most flamboyant patient in 2003 was the stockbroker Rene Rivkin, who had collapsed with a seizure on his first day in Silverwater Detention Centre. Charlie removed a meningioma, a common low-grade tumour, that was pressing against his temporal lobe and eroding the bone above his nose. He expected that some smaller growths would require future surgery. Cynics suspected a rich man's ruse to avoid his nine months of weekend detention for insider trading and questioned whether the tumour existed at all. But Rivkin had had a meningioma removed at St Vincent's Hospital almost twenty years earlier and, after his scans stayed clear for more than a decade, he had stopped having check-ups. It returned, as even so-called benign tumours can. Charlie believed Rivkin's poor judgement and lack of remorse about his actions – illegally trading shares, making the transaction on a mobile phone that could be traced, driving soon after surgery – were typical signs of tumours in the frontal lobe, which controls the higher psychological processes. Combined with his bipolar disorder, it created the volatile character who would kill himself two years later as his professional and private lives disintegrated.

Most patients, however, were of interest only to their own family. Michael Bartrom was a business journalist who had left behind his wife and children in New Zealand to put his life in Charlie's hands. A benign tumour that had set off an epileptic fit seventeen years earlier had turned malignant and was causing more frequent fits. During the biopsy in December 2002, the neurosurgeon in New Zealand had nicked the carotid artery, damaged a nerve and spent all his effort staunching the blood. Bartrom woke up paralysed down his left side and blind in his right eye and still had his tumour. His doctors said they couldn't do any more.

A friend had seen a New Zealand current affairs program about two other patients of the same neurosurgeon who had turned to Charlie. 'Is this Dr Teo a miracle worker?' asked the show's host, Paul Holmes. The neurosurgeon in New Zealand did not think so.

'I believe he's offering patients an operation they could have in New Zealand, paid for by the public health,' he told the interviewer. Yet, he wasn't offering the operation, and he argued that Charlie was selling his patients false hope. 'We can't beat this disease with surgery.'

Charlie replied: 'In the majority of cases, yes, we are delaying someone's death. But if they have quality of life, you're not delaying death, you're prolonging life.'

By chance, one of the men who had appeared on the program was at Prince of Wales the week Bartrom was there. Neil McKenzie was a sixty-year-old general practitioner who played banjo in a jazz band, and swam and ran every day until a seizure signalled his illness in 2001. The diagnosis after a biopsy was the worst possible: grade 4 glioblastoma in his right frontal lobe, and a likely six months to live. He noted wryly that his oncologist had charged him a hundred dollars for the news. McKenzie sold his practice and booked in for palliative radiotherapy. But before his appointment came up, he saw a television news item about a community in New Zealand that had raised money to send a child to Charlie Teo.

A week after looking at McKenzie's scans, Charlie removed his tumour. McKenzie felt like a new man, full of joy. He went back to work one day a week, recorded a CD with his band and played regular games of squash. When a scan showed the tumour was regrowing eighteen months later, Charlie removed it again. After two months, in January 2003, he was back for removal of necrotic tissue caused by radiotherapy, and again now.

'Nine out of twelve New Zealanders who have come to Charlie are still alive,' McKenzie told me on the phone from New Zealand a few weeks later. 'He has done one girl seven times and one man is alive eight years later. There are good papers proving that a radical approach, removing the whole thing, can extend life.'

He was appalled, though not surprised, at the criticism aimed at Charlie. 'When you get people rewriting the textbooks they are usually frowned on by society.' But when he thought about the treatment he'd had from his own profession, he said, 'I feel ashamed at being a doctor. You always have to put your patients first and put your ego behind you. When you get something like this thrown at you, hope is what you want.'

Charlie brought his daughters to the ward after McKenzie's surgery. He wrapped his arm around his patient, handed him a piece of healing crystal given to him by a Tibetan Buddhist monk, and asked the nurses, 'Does this look like a man with a brain tumour?' No one mentioned the word 'cure'. McKenzie was realistic about where he was headed. But he wasn't just marking time. He was living. When he went back to New Zealand, his mission was to lodge a complaint against the neurosurgeon who had tried to deny him that and to carry on living as long as possible. He had read about tests being done at American and British universities, using the diphtheria toxin as a treatment for brain tumours.

'I'm going for it,' he said. 'I'd like to be cured.'

Michael Bartrom, the other New Zealander, came out of his surgery looking like the loser in a heavyweight boxing fight – one eye closed, a limp arm and leg, head slashed, speech slurred – but no worse than when he'd gone in. In fact, for now, much better: an MRI showed no tumour in his brain and his fits had settled down.

Bartrom knew that removing a hundred per cent of his tumour did not remove the danger. A malignant tumour would grow back from the invisible cells left behind, doubling in size every six weeks. But he would go home, have radiotherapy and follow Charlie's advice: eat a diet rich in antioxidants, give up coffee, take evening primrose, exercise, meditate and stay positive. He would return to work as a journalist and enjoy each day with his wife and teenagers, knowing he had done all he could to stay alive for them.

'Coming here is like making a pilgrimage to Lourdes. It's a last resort. I've got a fighting chance now,' he said.

The worst thing his doctors had done to him was not the physical harm, nor their willingness to capitulate to his disease, but their refusal to refer him to Charlie, or even acknowledge a different style of treatment. Their attitude was not illegal but Bartrom considered it amoral.

'There's no excuse for not offering patients the best form of treatment available . . . When someone tells you to go home and look at the sunset, it's a losing game. The biggest thing Charlie offers is hope. This is established medical practice with well-documented proof behind it. You have to wonder why the medical community is ignoring it. It's their duty to offer the best medical opportunities and I see no reason why that shouldn't include sending you to another doctor.

'I have no vision of a future that doesn't include me,' he added with the clarity of a man ready for the next round.

Within a few days, Bartrom was on a plane to Auckland. All up, he had spent thirty thousand dollars on surgery and anaesthesia, and travel and accommodation for him and his father. He considered it a bargain. Four years later, he would still be alive and fighting.

Charlie had more good news that week in March 2003. He was a finalist in the New South Wales awards for Australian of the Year. The winner was Father Chris Riley, a Sydney-based minister who worked hard and selflessly with street kids. But Charlie was pleased to have public support because at the same time he was under more pressure than ever before within the profession.

The four Perth neurosurgeons whose young patients had gone to Charlie and attracted media coverage were still trying to have him deregistered two years later. They hadn't accepted Charlie's letter of apology. They complained that he had not communicated with them when treating their patients, which was the equivalent of 'stealing', and that he had used the media to criticise them and benefit his own career. They wanted him out of the profession.

Charlie's lawyer persuaded him to accept the complaint about communication, even though he knew communicating with the other surgeons was a matter of etiquette rather than a requirement. He didn't get much etiquette in return.

When he'd first returned from America, he had rung a colleague and said, 'I've just seen your patient for a second opinion and I think I can take that tumour out, especially if you say you can't. Would you mind if I do?' He could hear the sarcastic chill in the other surgeon's voice as he said, 'Yes, you can take it out, Charlie. Only you can take it out. No one else can do it.' In a similar situation, another surgeon had replied, 'Take the tumour out but tell the patient I won't see her again.'

Charlie said he would correspond with other neurosurgeons in every case if every other neurosurgeon in the country undertook to do the same. Likewise, he would ask permission to talk to the media if everyone else did so. He was adamant that he had not abused the surgeons to the media.

'I've never once badmouthed my colleagues,' he said. 'I don't say to my patients, "So-and-so has stuffed up" or "So-and-so is a bad neurosurgeon," because all they do is offer a different perspective. They have made a learned decision based on their own personal experience, their reading of the literature and their own personality, which might not be as positive as mine. What I am irate about is that they actually tell people not to come and see me.'

Charlie was just as determined as his enemies, so the argument dragged on for several years until it simply petered out. Meanwhile, his reputation had sprung another leak. His sense of humour had got him into trouble again.

At least one person had taken him seriously when, at the end of Aaron McMillan's operation, Charlie looked down at his sodden gown and joked, 'Look. I've pissed myself!' A complaint was made to the hospital that he had urinated on the floor of the theatre, a gross breach of surgical hygiene. The story was humiliating, damaging and wrong. The neurosurgeons David Kadrian and Peter Nakaji and others knew he'd just been playing around for the television camera. But the rumour spread so widely that a nurse who had nothing to do with Aaron's case wept at the horror of Charlie's misbehaviour. Once again, he had to defend himself against hostile inquisitors.

At home, Genevieve Teo was good-natured and adaptable.

She ran the house, was always there for the children, turned on dinners and all-night parties for Charlie's colleagues, and travelled with him whenever she could. Yet, naturally, she felt the strain of her husband's battles. She also shared the emotional impact of his patients' illnesses and worried about the effect on their children of living so close to the sick and dying. But she understood that Charlie felt honoured when someone flew across the country or the world to have him operate and that he couldn't just leave them alone in a hotel room. So she encouraged him to invite them out for a paddle in his kayak and welcomed them home for dinner. The liveliness of four little girls was a useful distraction.

Some doctors thought it was unethical and even dangerous to befriend patients when you had to make dispassionate decisions about their treatment, particularly when they might die. For Charlie, there was no fixed barrier. His three-year-old patient from Perth, Lily Glaskin, and her family had stayed with the Teos after her surgery. When she died after many months of surgery and other treatment, Charlie was angry with himself as he watched his daughters' tears and tried to explain the death of a little girl.

'Daddy, did Lily have a brain tumour?' asked his daughter Nikki from the back seat of their Suzuki four-wheel drive, one afternoon.

'Yes, she did.'

'So why didn't you fix it?'

'Because she didn't come to me first. She went to someone else and they didn't take the tumour out. If you don't take it out the first time, there's no chance of curing it.'

'So if she went to them first and then came to you and she died . . . ?'

'It doesn't make me look good, does it?'

Charlie didn't have the answers. Even with the best surgical skills, he couldn't win the race against brain cancer. Until researchers discovered the causes and ways to switch the tumours off, or at least improved the treatments, neurosurgeons were fighting a war with pop guns. Challenged on all fronts, he did not think about a retreat. Instead, he decided to join the search for a cure.

In March 2003, a month after Aaron's concert at the Sydney Opera House, Charlie put on his own gala event. The Cure for Life Foundation was launched with a ball and charity auction at the Australian Jockey Club, a few blocks from Prince of Wales Hospital, with the New South Wales Governor, Marie Bashir, as patron. Only four other neurosurgeons joined the crowd: Charlie's colleagues Bernie Kwok and Marcus Stoodley, and two surgeons from St George Hospital, Mark Davies and Erica Jacobsen, the latter of whom now had her own practice. The rest made their point by staying away. But a thousand people were there to celebrate what might one day be possible. Many were patients, still in the limbo of treatment, or former patients forever changed by their strange inward journey.

Vicki Hackett, a glamorous Qantas flight attendant, was in high spirits. Two years earlier, as a part-time psychology student, she was leaving a lecture on the pineal gland when a sudden partial seizure made her leg shake uncontrollably. A neurologist she found through the Yellow Pages diagnosed a tumour on her own pineal gland, which the French philosopher René Descartes pinpointed as the seat of consciousness, and modern medicine knows as the manufacturer of melatonin and controller of the body's circadian rhythms, a vulnerable function in flight crews.

'If there's one man who can remove this tumour,' said the neurologist, 'I know who it is.' Two days later, Charlie had the tumour out and told Hackett with a grin, 'I've operated on your soul.'

Since then, Hackett had ended an unhappy marriage, achieved a high distinction in a neuroanatomy exam and noticed that her sketches of African game animals were now more realistic. Despite the need for further surgery to drain fluid from her brain, with the tumour eradicated, she said, 'I would have felt worse if I'd been told I had to have a breast removed. It's a strange thing to say, but having a brain tumour is probably one of the best things that's ever happened to me because it resulted in so many improvements in my life and an appreciation of the here and now.'

Charlie, dressed in an elegant Mao-collared dinner suit, hosted the ball with ebullient goodwill. 'I'm not sure why I'm up here,' he said from the stage. 'It must be for my sexual prowess.' The evening was being filmed by the ABC for another episode of *Australian Story*, titled 'The Trouble with Charlie', which would open with him riding his motorbike to a soundtrack of Abba.

A laugh and a groan went around the room but the focus returned to his plea to raise a million dollars. With a ninety-five per cent cure rate for leukaemia, he said, brain cancer was now the number one cancer killer in children. It attacked adults in their prime, and the average life expectancy for a patient with a malignant tumour was no better than it was fifty years before. Government funding was limited. Charlie wanted to put researchers into a lab with access to the bank of tumour tissue he was collecting from patients.

Among the foundation trustees was Sharon Aaron, whose four-year-old daughter, Sara, had recently undergone an emergency operation for a peach-sized tumour pressing against her brain stem. No one suspected a brain tumour was causing the little girl to vomit until she had a brain scan. Sara was well again by the night of the ball, though she would need another operation and therapy to regain her coordination. Her parents were dedicated to fundraising for children's rehabilitation.

'We felt like our whole life collapsed,' Sharon Aaron told me. 'We were putting our child's life in Charlie's hands. Had I known as much about him as I do now, I would have felt much better. He is incredibly gifted.'

Aaron McMillan had also joined the foundation as a board member and ambassador. After Charlie, he was the main speaker of the night. Leaning a hand on each side of the podium, he said, 'I take the responsibility of being a successful long-term survivor very, very seriously. As Charlie recently said to me, "There just aren't many of you around."'

He thanked Charlie not only for saving his life eighteen months earlier, but for opening up a new world of music even as he had lain on the operating table. 'Last time I visited him at home, he played me the four-CD set of the complete John Denver collection . . . and somehow they all seemed familiar.'

Aaron was also part of the night's entertainment, playing a grand piano in the centre of the ballroom. But his greatest contribution to the event's success was the last act. When Tim Farriss raked his guitar strings and INXS began blasting their old hits through the speakers, the night was given over to dancing. The ball raised almost a quarter of a million dollars. The most hotly contested prize among the luxuries up for auction was a working trip with Charlie to Peru and a trek up to Machu Picchu. Two people bid so furiously that each was granted the prize for forty thousand dollars. Kerry Armstrong, an actor who had seen the child of a friend saved by Charlie, was a passionate spokeswoman for the foundation. But even Charlie knew she'd gone too far that night when she said from the stage, 'He's controversial . . . But then, you know, so was Jesus.'

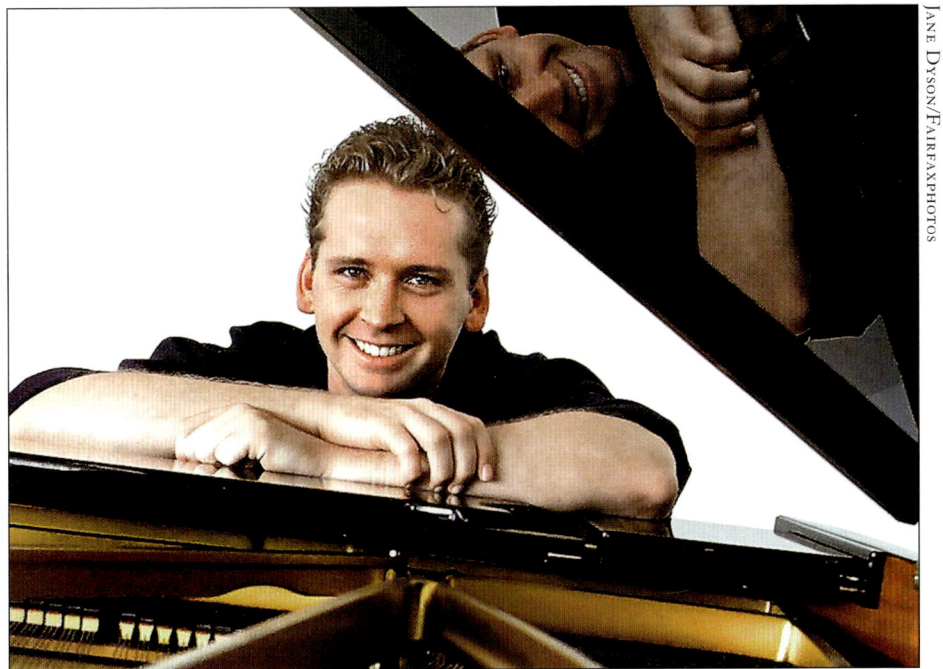

Jane Dyson/Fairfaxphotos

In February 2003, eighteen months after surgery for a brain tumour, Aaron McMillan was glowing with health and ambition as he rehearsed for his first solo concert at the Sydney Opera House.

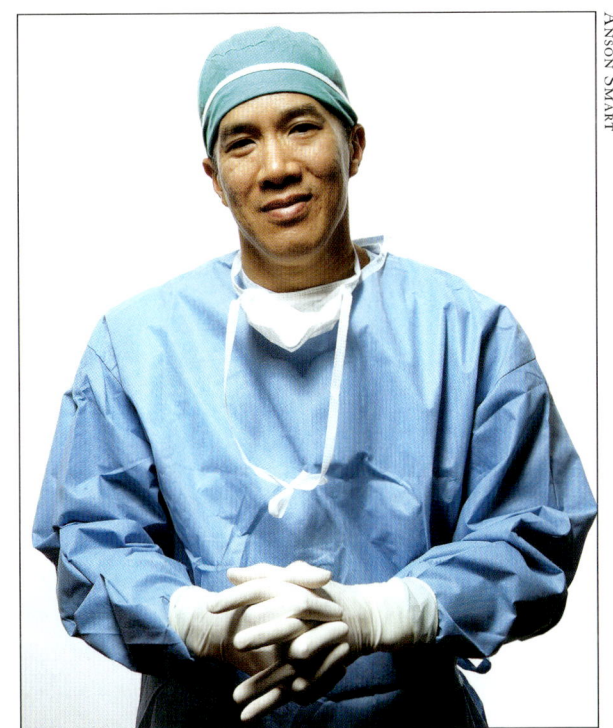

Anson Smart

Charlie Teo was at the peak of his career in 2007, at the age of forty-nine, with constant demand for his skills as a neurosurgeon from hospitals, universities and charities around the world.

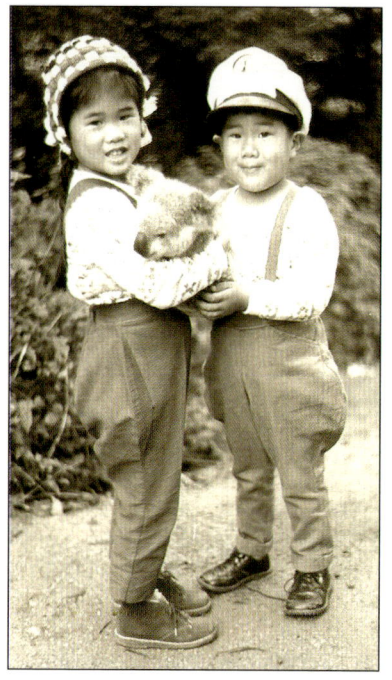
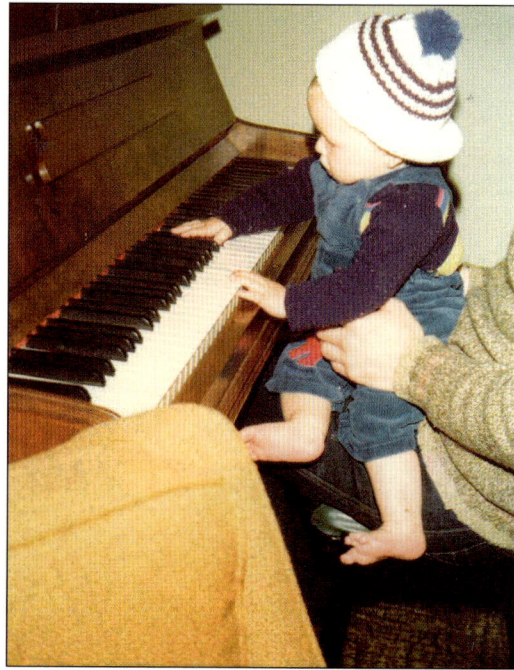

Left: In 1960, Charlie and his sister, Anne, were dressed like British royalty and introduced to Australian wildlife. *Right:* Aaron played his first notes in 1977 at the age of seven months, sitting on his uncle Mark Robinson's lap.

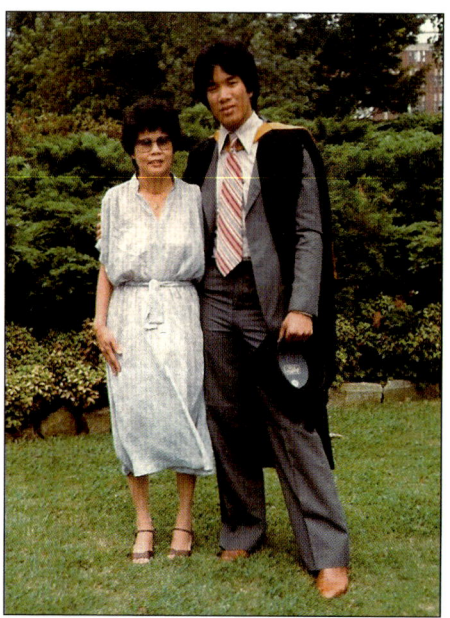
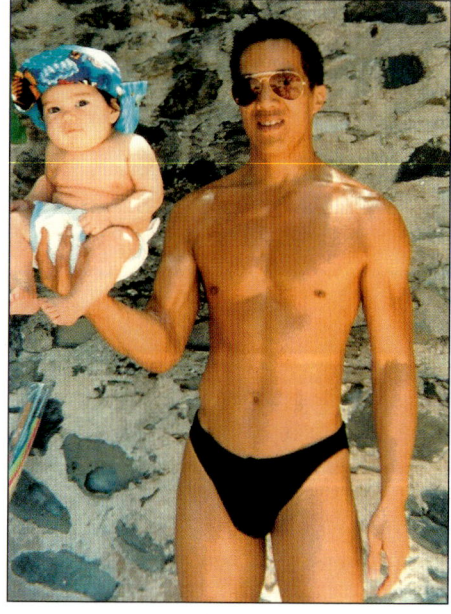

Left: The medical student with his mother, Elizabeth Teo, at his graduation from the University of New South Wales in 1981. *Right:* Father and eldest daughter, Alexandra, on holiday in Hawaii in 1992 before Charlie began work in Little Rock, Arkansas.

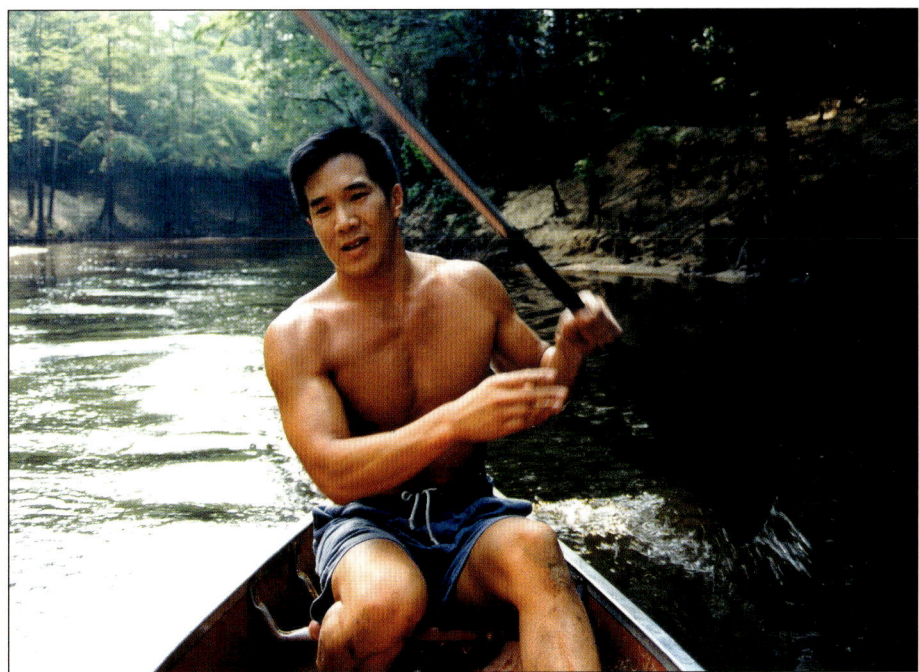

Always a competitive athlete, Charlie paddled his kayak on the Lane Cove River in Sydney in 1989, and still kayaks for fitness and relaxation.

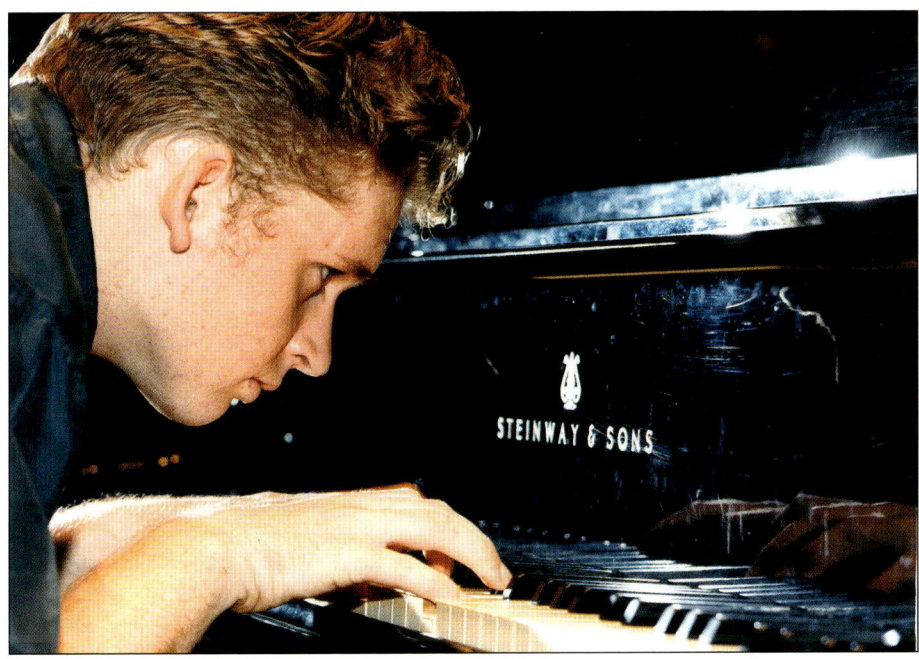

By the age of seventeen, Aaron was a full-time pianist and entrepreneur, organising concerts for himself and other musicians.

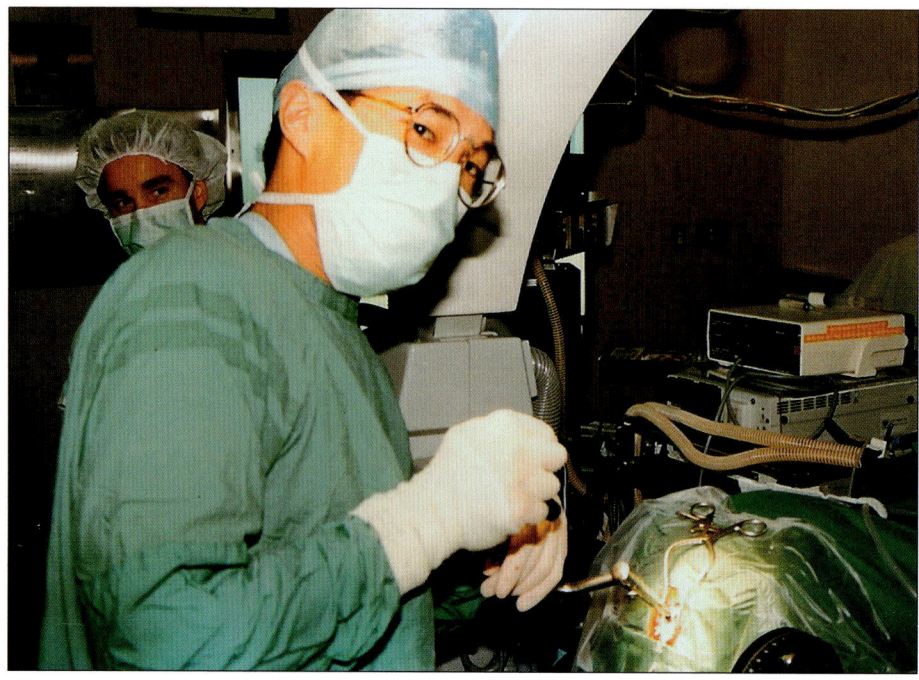

The young registrar in 1987 at Sydney's Royal Prince Alfred Hospital operating to save the life of a trauma victim with severe head injuries.

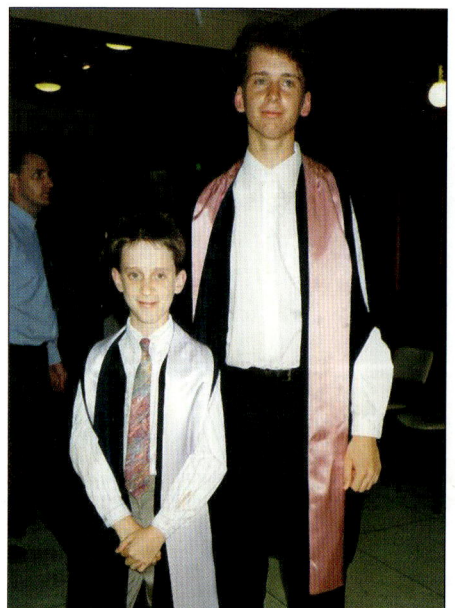
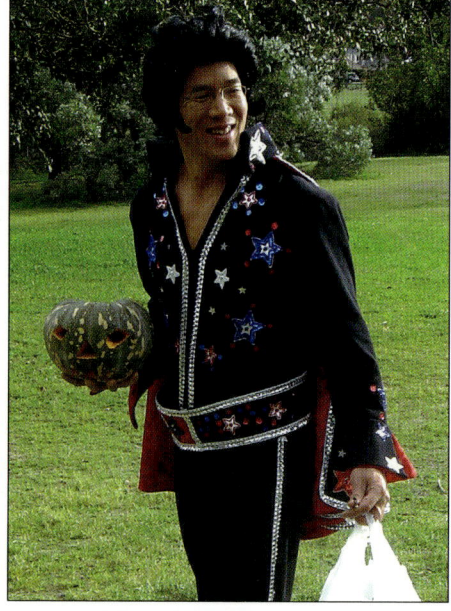

Left: In 1994, at the the age of sixteen, Aaron received his Licentiate Diploma of Music at the Sydney Conservatorium, alongside twelve-year-old Simon Tedeschi. *Right:* Charlie dressed as his musical hero Elvis Presley for his daughter's Halloween party in 2003.

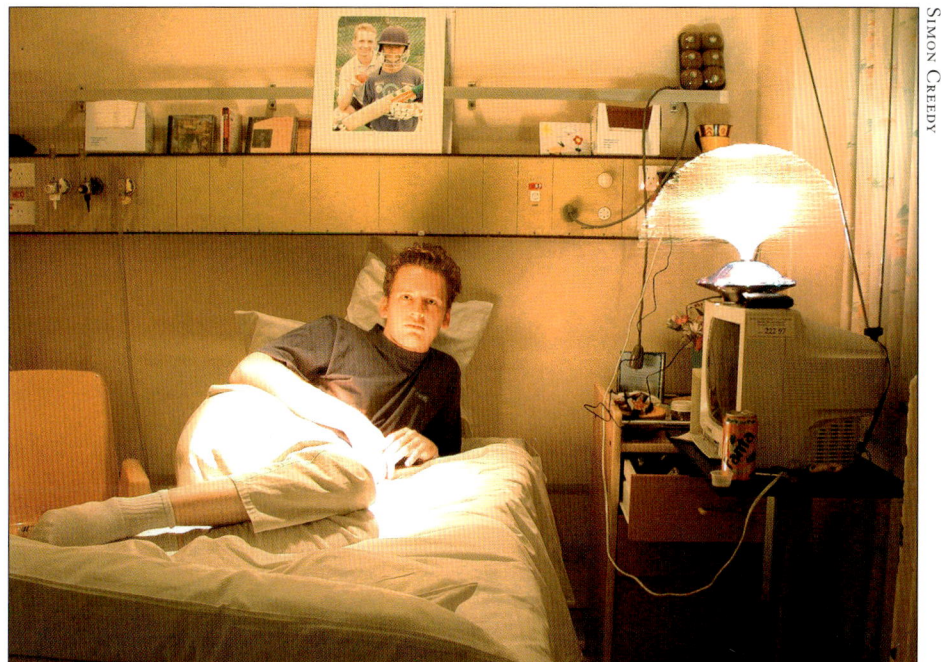

Aaron spent almost a month at Prince of Wales Hospital in 2001 while waiting for brain surgery. His ward became home, filled with friends, music and gifts.

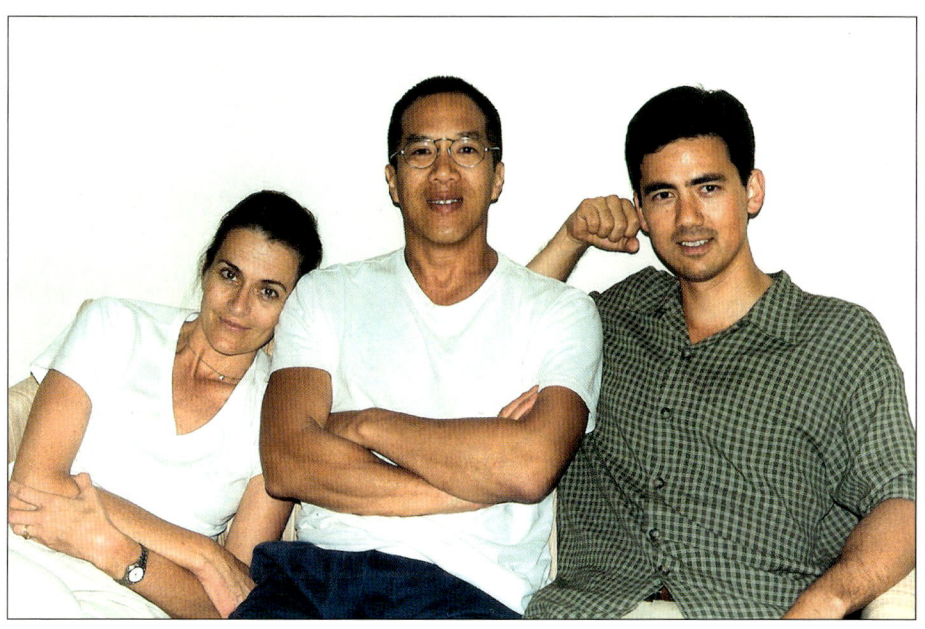

The year 2001 was intense for Charlie, pictured here with his wife, Genevieve, and Peter Nakaji, the American neurosurgeon who assisted on Aaron's operation while working with Charlie as a visiting fellow.

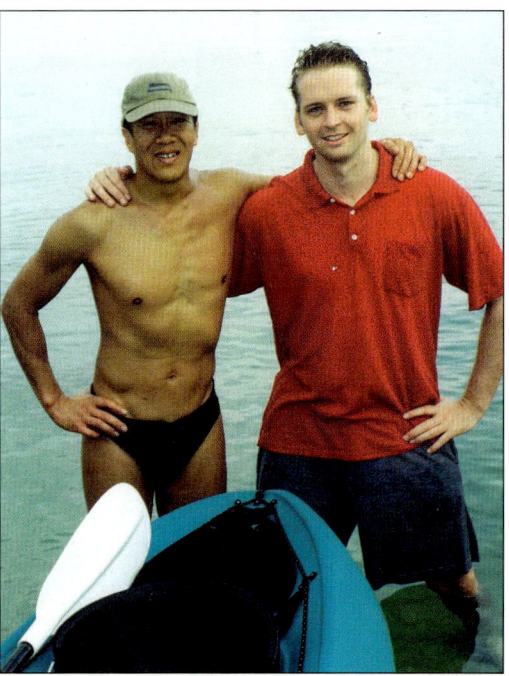
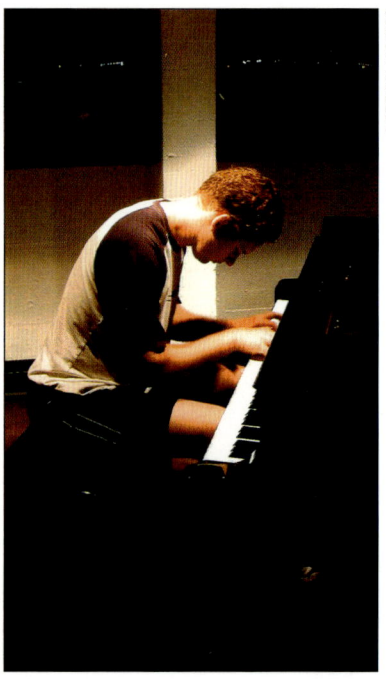

Left: Soon after Aaron's surgery in 2001, Charlie invited him to go kayaking on Sydney Harbour. *Right:* By early 2003, Aaron was practising on a new Steinway piano at the Sydney Opera House for a solo performance in the Concert Hall.

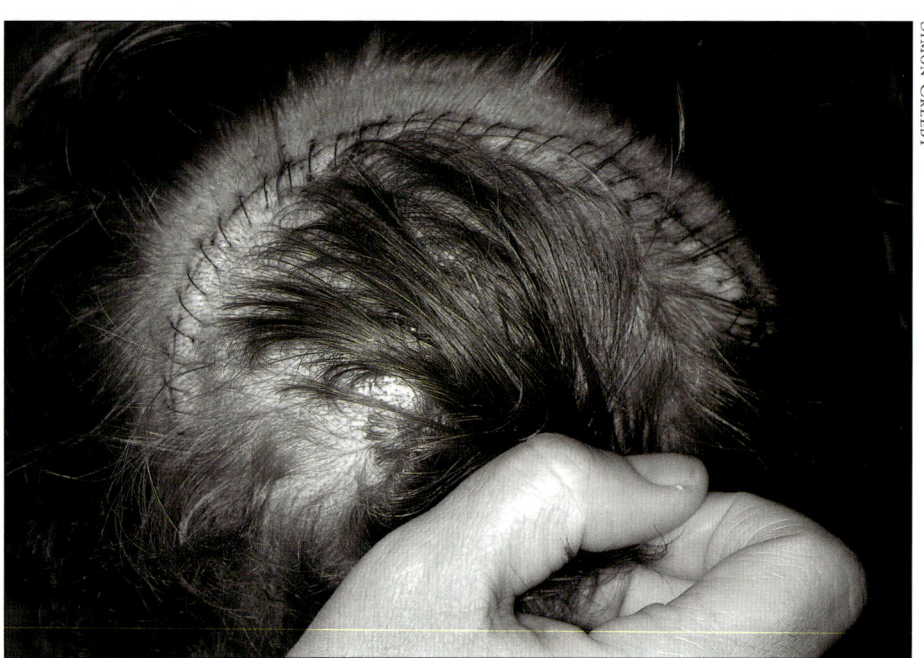

Charlie's neat needlework left Aaron with a minimal scar and most of his hair — important for a patient's healing and morale.

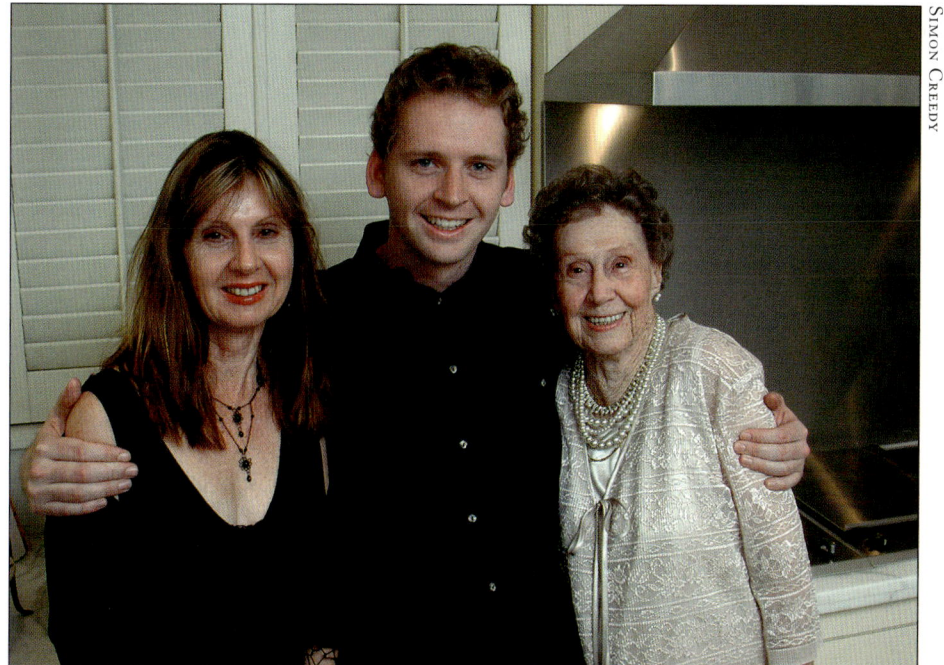

At a party in 2002 for the twelve-month anniversary of his operation, Aaron is pictured here with the two women he loved — his mother, Gail Puckett, and his grandmother, Marjorie Robinson.

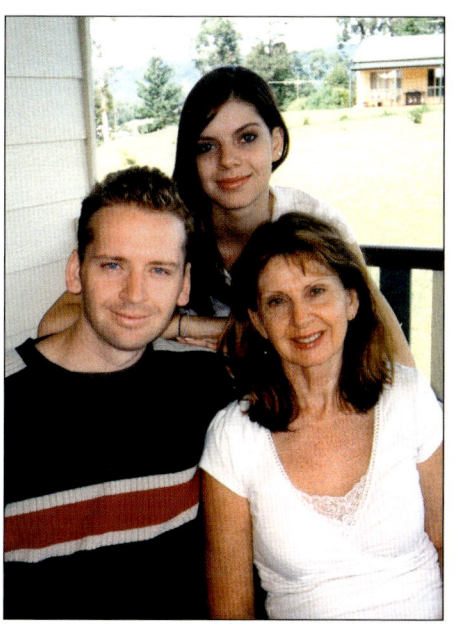

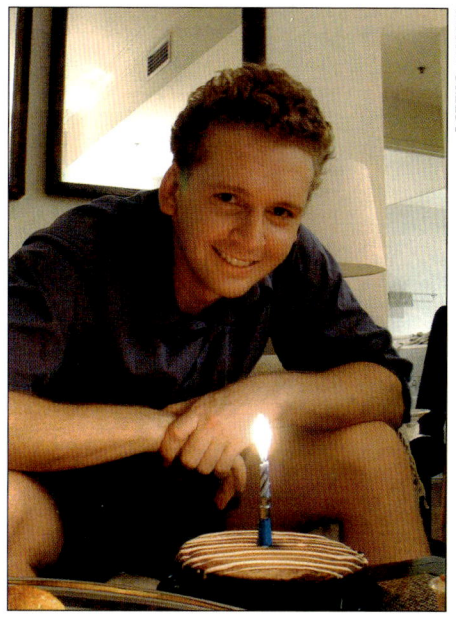

Left: A summer holiday in Brisbane at the end of 2003 with his mother and his sister, Amy. *Right:* Aaron took a break from preparations for his Opera House concert in February 2003 to celebrate his twenty-sixth birthday.

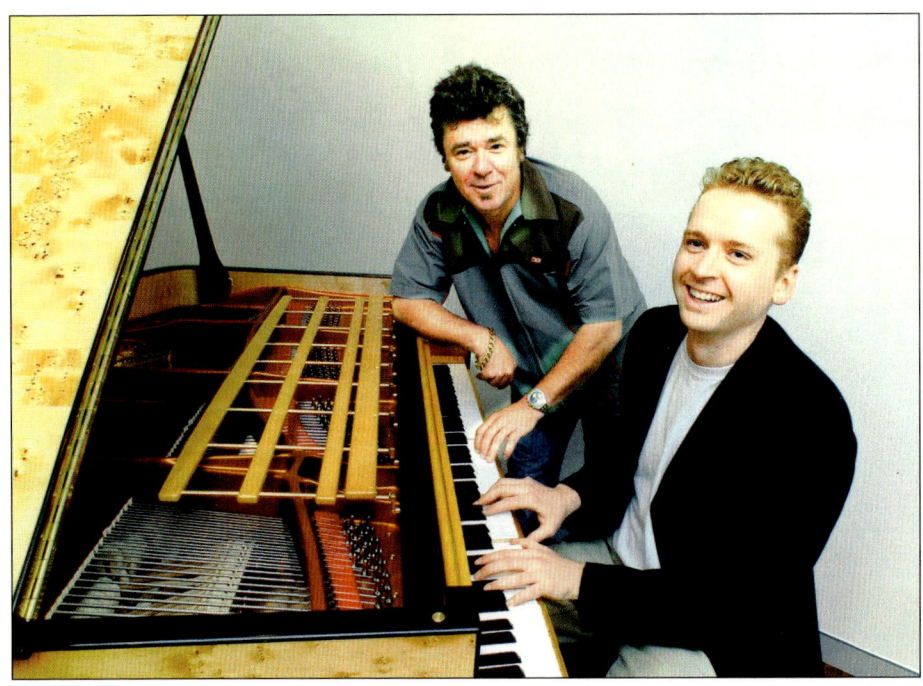

Aaron had a visit from his friend Tim Farriss of the band INXS during practice on an Australian-made Stuart piano for his 2004 Opera House concert of Australian music.

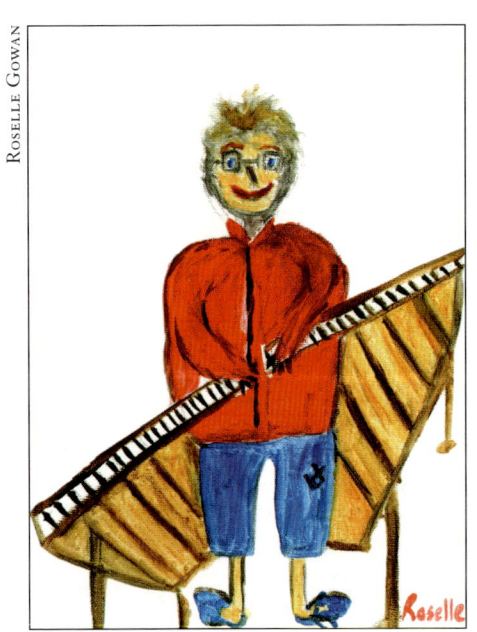

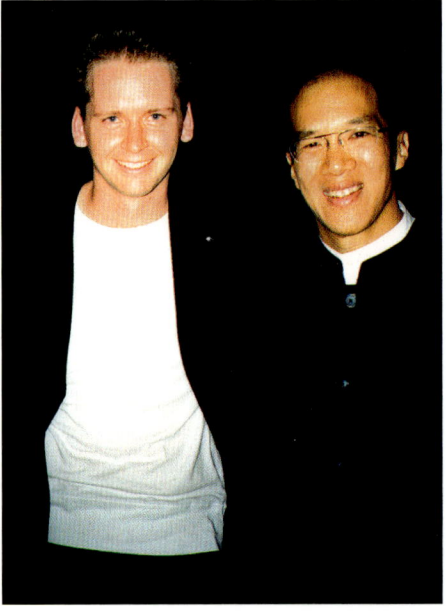

Left: Roselle Gowan captured her friend's boyishness in her 2007 painting *Master McMillan — Stepping Beyond Music*. *Right:* Aaron and Charlie at the fundraising ball to launch the Cure for Life Foundation in March 2003.

PART THREE

'The Chinese hold that if you save a man's life, you become responsible for him.'

Shirley Hazzard, *The Great Fire*

21

SHRAPNEL

Around midnight on 31 March 2003, Aaron took the lift down to the lobby of his apartment building carrying a pair of rubber gloves, a bucket and a spray bottle of cleaning fluid. Carefully, he fitted the gloves onto the extended hands of the nude marble statue that stood near the entrance, then hung the bucket over her wrist and stood the bottle at her feet. She was his April Fools' Day gift to the neighbours. It was a spontaneous joke, the kind of game Aaron and his friends frequently played with each other. The concierge smiled and pretended not to see. Next morning, the residents had no trouble guessing which exuberant neighbour had dressed their nymph.

Aaron slept late and spent the afternoon at his piano, occasionally gazing at the harbour view. He fantasised about owning the penthouse in the building but, thanks to a neighbour who gave him cheap rent, he was able to live in this small, elegant apartment, which was slowly accumulating the CDs, music scores, chocolate wrappers and other detritus of a young man's life.

'You can't get a more yellow key than D,' he told me as he played the familiar notes of Rachmaninov's Prelude in D.

Most ears could not 'hear' any yellow, but for Aaron every piece of music conjured a distinct band of the colour spectrum. He was certain he did not have the neurological condition synaesthesia, which blurs the senses, causing people to taste names or smell colours or see sounds; he simply associated each musical key and its mood with a colour. C major was pure white and the other keys fanned out in a rainbow from red A up to violet G. If he were asked to compose while sitting in a green field, for example, he knew he would have to write in grassy E flat or the more stridently green E. This was his personal interpretation but he was satisfied to learn that the Russian composer Alexander Scriabin had also linked each key with a colour. Aaron was un-comprehending when another composer told him he pictured G as the green key. G could only be violet.

In his imagination, he was starting to hear the sounds he wanted to use in his first really original music. He read books about the principles of composition and listened to African music. There was other groundwork to do for the leaps he hoped to make. He talked to the United Nations representative in Australia, Juan Carlos Brandt, about his vision for a world music organisation, and plotted out the Wayfarer website, which would be a platform to publicise first his work and then that of other musicians. There was an album of Australian music he had begun recording, and, as always, there were bills to pay.

Staying fit was not to be treated as a luxury anymore. He swam in the residents' pool and walked the quiet streets late at night, skirting the tourist hangouts of The Rocks. Sometimes he did a coaching session with Elliot Bullock, who was finishing school and planning his cricket career. He had also begun mentoring a young rock band he'd met through his family in Brisbane, a bunch of schoolboys who had talent but not much discipline. Aaron saw his teenage self in their bright faces and told them they could be the next INXS if they cared enough.

But, as the months went by, he couldn't shake off a lingering fatigue and sometimes complained of a dull pain and crunching sound in his jaw. Friends noticed that he opened and closed his mouth like a fish and massaged his right cheek as if to loosen a tightness there. Aaron dismissed it as an after-effect of his operation and having his head held in a clamp, face down, for fourteen hours. Perhaps it was just tension.

'Charlie,' I said tentatively as we bounced along in his four-wheel drive one Friday afternoon in mid-2003, when it was his turn to pick up the girls from school, 'is there any chance Aaron's pain could be related to his tumour?'

'It's possible,' said Charlie. 'But the temptation when you've had a tumour is to suspect every little pain is related.'

A dentist saw nothing he could treat and sent Aaron to a chiropractor who specialised in jaws. Feeling some relief after the first manipulation, he went back for a second. That night, he threw up. The next morning, he felt as if he had been mugged. Unable to lift or turn his head, he was virtually paralysed by the pain in his neck. The chiropractor made a home visit the next day but with the lightest touch to Aaron's neck, he risked a punch in the face. He could only suggest rest to let the disturbance settle.

No better a week later, Aaron went once again to Prince of Wales Hospital in an ambulance; sitting in a car was impossible. An X-ray showed no damage, so the staff sent him home with painkillers that at least enabled him to stand. But after another week of pain, he rang Charlie.

'Something's really, really wrong,' he said.

An MRI showed nothing, and before Charlie left for a conference in Italy he tried to comfort Aaron by telling him he was a big wuss. But he was puzzled and concerned. He consulted his colleague Shaun Watson, a neurologist who worked both at Prince of Wales and at a practice in Blacktown in western Sydney. They shared rooms, and often patients suffering from headaches or epilepsy. Watson, just turned forty, had been one of the younger neurologists in the crowd gathered at Prince of Wales when Aaron put on the show before his surgery. He remembered the young man's confident account of his symptoms and the hum of curiosity in the room. He had also been one of the few doctors at the Cure for Life Foundation launch, where he was moved by Aaron's performance.

Watson had chosen neurology because it retained a beautiful simplicity in the age of high-tech medicine. Ninety per cent of its art was in talking to patients and examining them for symptoms. It was more contemplative and less interventionist than neurosurgery, relying mostly on drugs, rehabilitation and reassurance. When further tests were needed, advances in technology kept improving diagnosis.

But Aaron and a new set of brain scans mystified him. No abnormality showed. 'There must be a mechanical problem,' he thought, 'a severe version of the common cricked neck, perhaps triggered by the chiropractic treatment.' He advised Aaron to have a bone scan, which would begin with an injection of radioactive dye, hopefully showing up any trauma.

With a neck brace and lots of pills, Aaron was able to hobble about at home and work on his computer in bed. 'January turned into December for me this year,' he said in frustration as 2003 rushed to an end. By then, although he still couldn't turn his head, he told himself and his doctors he was improving. He put off the bone scan, and spent a quiet Christmas and New Year with his family in Brisbane, hoping relaxation would speed his recovery. He walked on the beach, ate his mother's food and hung out with the kids – his brother and sister, the band members, and a few of his mother's pupils. Instead of feeling better, though, he noticed the right side of his tongue was becoming weak and a slight lisp slurred his speech. His right shoulder had dropped, tilting his head to the left, and he'd developed a sharp pain in his fifth rib.

A little frightened, he rang Shaun Watson from the Central Coast of New South Wales, where he'd gone to visit his grandparents at their new retirement unit. All weekend, for distraction, Aaron had kept himself busy cataloguing his grandparents' classical music CDs in chronological order and listening to the first nineteen recordings. He finished with Beethoven. He wanted his music to be as good as the young Beethoven's; mature Beethoven was unmatchable.

The neurologist was shocked by what he heard. The weakness in Aaron's tongue sounded sinister and he seemed to have fractured a rib simply by rolling over in bed. Watson sent him for an immediate bone scan at Nepean Hospital and then summoned him to his rooms at Blacktown. Based on what he saw on the scan – a small irregularity in the neck and a 'hot spot' in the rib – Watson ordered another, urgent, MRI covering the area from the top of his neck to his brain.

It was 9 January 2004, a blazing hot Friday when most of Sydney was still on holidays and the first bushfires of the season were closing in on the city's northern suburbs. After an exhausting day of scans, Aaron drove into Sydney. The lease on his apartment had run out and he was planning to find a new place after the holidays but, meanwhile, he was homeless, so he arranged to drop in on his friend Simon Creedy while waiting for the results from Watson. When Simon's phone rang late in the afternoon, it was Charlie, just back from his summer holiday in Perth. He commanded Aaron over to his rooms.

Fear vibrated through Aaron's body as he drove up the familiar Randwick street to the hospital, walked the long corridor and caught the lift to the pink office on the seventh floor. He had spent months assuring himself he had an injury that would eventually take care of itself. Now Charlie was looking through the pile of scans and dipping into his lolly jar and saying the words Aaron had dreaded.

'Oh, fuck. There's something there.'

Among the two hundred images, just four showed a strange shadow that looked like two cherries joined by a stem in the back of Aaron's neck.

'Could they be cysts, or blood clots caused by the chiropractor?' Aaron asked.

'That would be the best possible outcome,' Charlie said. The worst outcome would be that it was a new type of cancer and he'd be dead in two weeks, or he might have chemotherapy and live for five months. Charlie was half joking, using the shock to help Aaron absorb the bad news. It was a tumour, he knew that much, but it didn't look like a recurrence of the old one. Thinking aloud, he said he might be able to resect it and fuse the vertebrae at the top of Aaron's neck if they were badly damaged. But, again, that would most likely ruin his piano playing. Radiotherapy was the alternative and not a great one.

'I think I'm an angel sent down to test your skills,' Aaron said.

Charlie was more upset than he let Aaron see and his weekend wasn't going to get any better. His next-door neighbour had died from melanoma after a long illness. Matthew Fiddick, a fourteen-year-old Perth boy whose case had been covered by SBS television for a series on inspirational stories, was back in hospital. Charlie had operated on him five times over many years and he had shown extraordinary spirit. His tumour was an ependymoma, which had been partly removed by another doctor and followed with radiotherapy, but remaining tumours had turned malignant and were regrowing every six weeks, causing gradual nerve damage and paralysis.

Back in Ward 8 at Prince of Wales three days later, Aaron had had another round of CT scans and was in a bed very close to where he had lain two and a half years earlier, except the renovated room had been painted in cheerful kindergarten colours. Dressed in shorts and a Rip Curl T-shirt, his long legs dangling off the bed, he seemed poised to leave. Brian McMillan sat quietly in a chair.

Charlie whirled in at 7.30 pm, looking like a kung-fu star with his freshly shaven head. He'd had a dark day: an old friend had come in with a brain tumour and even Charlie had advised against operating.

A southerly was blowing away another scorcher. Later, there would be lightning, thunder and rain. The wind moaned through a slit of open window as Charlie sat for ten long minutes going through the new set of scans. He sighed once then pulled his chair to the end of the bed. Aaron was struggling to open a bag of mints and Charlie took it, ripped it apart and tossed one in his mouth. He spoke around the bulge in his cheek.

'It isn't good.'

The shadow on the scans was a tumour that had eroded the base of Aaron's skull. Charlie would be talking to specialists in radiotherapy and chemotherapy the next day, although chemo-therapy was known to be ineffective on secondary tumours from a hemangiopericytoma.

In 2001, Charlie had made the difficult decision not to follow Aaron's operation with radiotherapy treatment. While it might have destroyed any invisible rogue cells from the tumour, it would also have damaged the healthy brain tissue. It could prolong the lives of patients with malignant tumours but it could also cause long-term lethargy, memory loss, hormonal disturbance, as well as new tumours or radiation necrosis, where brain cells began dying months or years later. Once again, Charlie had considered the fact that even the slightest loss of mental or physical function would end Aaron's musical career. He had examined the literature from previous cases and judged that after such a clean resection and with close surveillance, the risk was worth taking.

As a younger doctor in America, he had tended to prescribe radiotherapy after surgery on a hemangiopericytoma, but the chairman of his neurosurgery department in Arkansas, Ossama Al-Mefty, had results that convinced him patients survived just as long without a recurrence if they didn't have radiotherapy. He had proved that himself; as far as he knew, he had never had a patient with a hemangiopericytoma that metastasised. His one other Australian patient with the same kind of tumour had required radiotherapy because the original tumour was attached to his carotid artery and could not be completely removed; as a result, he had partly lost his vision. Statistics didn't save lives, though. Charlie wasn't so sure now that he'd done the right thing for Aaron but he still couldn't think of a better strategy.

'In my defence,' he said, 'it was probably in your blood stream even when I operated.'

Aaron asked the question that was slinking around the walls. 'Am I likely to die in the next month?'

'No, and not in the next two years ... Look at Lance Armstrong.' Charlie pointed to the book on the bed, a memoir by the champion cyclist, who had recovered from testicular and secondary cancers and gone on to win the Tour de France seven consecutive times. 'Anyway, I need you for the foundation,' he added.

'Should I keep working at my music?' Aaron asked.

Charlie answered without hesitation. 'Tell yourself you want to play at a concert or get to your tenth school reunion.'

'Can we make that my fiftieth reunion?'

Charlie left to visit Matthew Fiddick, who was fading as his brain stem function failed, decreasing his ability to swallow or breathe. Aaron and Brian discussed Charlie's words. They grasped at the assurance that Aaron would not die in the next two years. Numbers had a seductive and dangerous power, as Aaron had learned: his first death sentence had been 'six weeks'. Right now, two years seemed like forever. Surely a cure would emerge before then.

22

IT'S RAINING IN TAMWORTH

A new phase of treatment began, bringing full-body scans and Dr Bob Smee, a radiation oncologist with a grey moustache, a gruff laugh and a sub-specialisation in brain tumours. He and Charlie respected one another's skills even though each found the other stubbornly attached to his own methods. They were in agreement over Aaron, however. His widespread cancer was inoperable and chemotherapy had proved ineffective in similar cases. Radiotherapy was the only option.

Charlie spent a night studying the literature and speaking to colleagues in Sydney and France. He learned that the mean survival time was forty-eight months after developing second-aries from hemangiopericytoma. Some people barely made two months, but at least one had lived on for twenty years.

Aaron was in a sweaty panic as he sat in a tiny, airless room a few days after his admission, waiting for a reading of his new scans. He had been peppered with bullets: there were five cancers in his neck, rib, hip and spine, and a spot – 'half the size of a pea,' he said – at the back of his brain. But Charlie thought that might be an enlarged blood vessel and no one else mentioned it.

Smee tried to be positive. He had a patient with the same kind of cancer who returned every couple of years for radiotherapy and then went on with his normal life. Aaron liked that story but he had to ask The Question.

'Do you expect me to be around in five years?'

Smee paused. 'No, I don't think so. But I'm frequently wrong and I don't mind being proved wrong.'

Aaron rejected an offer of prescription painkillers. His rib was aching but he remembered how dependent he'd become on dexamethasone and wanted to stay clear-headed. He would control his pain with meditation. He rang Charlie to ask if over-the-counter medication was all right. Sure, said Charlie from a room at a city hotel. Somehow he had locked away the grief of his recent working days and was celebrating his fifteenth wedding anniversary with Genevieve.

When a cluster of registrars gathered round Aaron's bed in the morning, he braced himself and said, 'Before you say anything, I want each of you to give me some good news.'

They did what they were told.

'It's raining in Tamworth,' one of them adlibbed.

'You don't have a tumour in your nose,' said another.

As Sydney sizzled through February, Aaron sizzled through twenty days of radiotherapy. Strapped onto the treatment bed with a specially moulded mask holding his face motionless, he looked like a futuristic warrior. An invisible beam hit his neck in a computer-outlined area that precisely matched the shape of the tumour. After eight seconds, the machine swung around to another position and then another, seven times, so that it penetrated the tumour from different angles without overdosing the surrounding flesh or the delicate spinal cord and brain. Multileaf collimation was a greatly refined version of the old lead blocks used to protect patients' vital organs from X-rays. Prince of Wales had been using the technique for four years and was still the only Australian hospital that offered it.

Under his mask, Aaron pretended he was having his photograph taken; he heard a buzzing noise but felt nothing except a slight tingling after a few days. As the treatment went on and the tumour shrank, he could move his neck more freely.

His file was marked 'palliative' – that modern euphemism that sounds gentle but that we know means care for the incurable. How could all the expensive equipment be no more than a Band-Aid? How could the doctors and nurses do their job every day if they thought it was futile? And who had decided Aaron couldn't be cured? He certainly hadn't.

Bob Smee met me at the cafe opposite Prince of Wales, where Aaron had filled in time before his surgery with coffee and cakes. He wore his twenty years of experience with visible weariness, and his friendliness suggested it was a relief to talk. I wanted to know if he was able to cure any of the fifty or sixty patients he saw every day.

'Of course, of course!' he said with a reassuring grin.

But his answer was qualified. A lot of his work ended up being palliative, patching people up rather than saving them. The luckier ones moved into a heavily populated grey zone.

'If a patient doesn't have any more problems with a tumour, even though it's still there, is that a cure? Or is the only definition of a cure that it's gone, it's been removed? If that's the case, then I don't necessarily cure a lot of people. If the criterion is they go on and live many, many years and they never have any more problems, then there are cures.'

Aaron was one of only three people he'd treated with hemangiopericytoma in the past five years from a total of about three thousand patients. The disease had metastasised in one other, a man in his thirties – the patient Smee had mentioned to Aaron – but, seven years later, he was still living normally and dropping in for occasional radiotherapy.

If there were to be any criticism of the way Charlie had handled Aaron's case, it would come from a sceptic like Smee. But he was adamant that Charlie had done nothing wrong.

'Absolutely not. Aaron can play the piano as a consequence of Charlie's surgery. Aaron's quality of life is better, his quantity of life is better. The nature of his tumour has nothing to do with the surgery. It metastasised in a microscopic fashion. When I met him, he'd had neck pain for six months and he'd had imaging four or five months prior to presentation and that imaging was clear, but there was obviously microscopic disease there.'

Radiotherapy had advanced since Smee was a young doctor but outcomes weren't always better. Each time Aaron went in for his brief session under the rays, the health system was charged up to three thousand dollars. The real cost was closer to ten thousand. Smee was also dispirited by the slowness of bureaucracy. He was trying to get approval from the New South Wales Health Department for a new version of the machine that treated Aaron, but he didn't like his chances.

The only way Smee could do his job was by detaching himself emotionally from each patient as he moved on to the next. Maybe that ability was in his nature, or maybe he had become better at it over time. It could make him seem cold. Sometimes he kicked himself for thoughtless things he did or said to patients. Perhaps he shouldn't have answered Aaron's 'five years' question so frankly.

'I'm not as hard-hearted as I sound,' he said, a smile hiding beneath his moustache.

Aaron's vitality and optimism impressed him, but he wouldn't go as far as Charlie did in accepting the influence of the mind on the body.

'Those who are positive certainly live better but there's not a lot of scientific evidence that they live longer. They are more likely to be at peace. They are less likely to be angry at their disease. They're more likely to be functioning in life instead of agitating and treading water.'

Aaron was trying to get on with his life. He had moved in with his aunt, Dene McMillan, at Bondi and she drove him to the hospital each morning on the way to her job as a high school history and English teacher. With its well-worn furniture and Asian objects, her flat was more bohemian than the luxurious eyries overlooking the harbour that Aaron was used to, and it sat above the rocks at a wild point called Ben Buckler, where the surf roared and the spray hit the windows. Aaron had space and company, and no rent to pay. There was even a piano in the living room.

Walking along the sand with friends was restorative. Among them was Anna Parsch, an old school friend who had qualified as a doctor and was planning to work overseas. A pretty woman with an upbeat spirit, she helped Aaron remember the pleasures of being a young man. They hadn't seen much of each other since their schooldays, but she had visited him in hospital before his surgery and strolled with him on Coogee beach. Her company had a calming effect and their childhood reminiscences helped him step outside the anxious present. She had since broken up with her boyfriend and a little flame of attraction flickered in Aaron. Impossible, maybe, but it was more fun to dwell on than radiotherapy. There was no doubt he was alive.

23

Travel at the Speed of Thought

Aaron's twenty-seventh birthday, 11 February 2004, fell in the middle of his radiotherapy treatment, but rather than languishing, he hired a catamaran and invited his family and friends to cruise around Sydney Harbour for the evening. He played keyboard and introduced the night's entertainment, which included a talented eight-year-old violinist called Alison Laurens, and ended with Indicator, the Queensland band Aaron mentored, jamming as he cut into a huge birthday cake. Apart from his stiff neck and crooked shoulder, he looked well enough to dispel his guests' most immediate fears.

Two weeks later, Sylvie Renaud-Calmel visited Aaron at his aunt Dene's Bondi flat, and he sat down at the piano to breeze through a Chopin waltz for her. He laughed at himself as he bungled the beginning two or three times.

'Oh, God,' he said, 'I must be tired.'

He concentrated and started again. The sound was completely

discordant and he realised his left hand was hitting the wrong keys. He knew the piece so well that there shouldn't have been a slip. He looked down and thought, 'I can't play, I can't see, I don't know where my hands are.' His left hand was disappearing off his mental screen and the octaves were overlapping in his mind. He could play the left-hand part with his right hand but he couldn't put the two parts together.

In a quiet panic, he sent Sylvie home and went to bed. A white light was flashing in his left peripheral vision and the only way to shut it out was to sleep. Next morning, it was still flickering and he was walking into walls on his left side, so he rang Charlie.

'You're about to have a seizure,' said Charlie. 'Come into Emergency.'

Over the next six days, Aaron had another series of brain scans and was put into a wired helmet for an electroencephalogram that drew the activity of his brain as a line of dramatic peaks and troughs. All the time he could see the white strobe light and the EEG registered electrical storm activity that showed he was having seizures right through the procedure. The staff had never seen that before. But nothing else seemed to be wrong. An MRI showed no regrowth of the brain tumour, no stroke, no other blockage to the blood vessels. Aaron suggested the radiotherapy may have disturbed his brain but the doctors dismissed that as impossible. Perhaps some scarring from his operation was causing the problem; there were cases where seizures had occurred ten or twenty years after surgery. Despite their unnerving effect, Shaun Watson pronounced the seizures 'partial' rather than life-threatening, and put him on a low dose of epilepsy medication. Charlie suggested an aspirin a day.

Aaron still believed that his fate wasn't just in the hands of doctors, who might be skilful but had shown they weren't omnipotent. In the end, he decided that he had to save himself. The scrutiny of his brain hadn't convinced him that that was all there was to him. As he put it, 'The brain for me is the physical stuff, whereas the mind and spirit is the thing that lives within us and uses that stuff.'

Friends and strangers alike all had a sure-fire alternative therapy to recommend, so Aaron agreed to try a treatment if three people spoke well of it. One such treatment was a mental healing therapy called The Journey, established by an American woman, Brandon Bays, who said she had healed herself of a large uterine tumour by eradicating old and troubling emotions. It was the same kind of lesson Brian tried to impart to Aaron through meditation.

Back on the ward, Aaron contacted a Journey therapist and had two sessions with her as he lay in bed. After guiding him into a deep meditation, she asked him to imagine travelling through his body and visiting the sites of his cancer. In his mental image, each spot appeared like a boulder towering over him. As he reached out to touch the cancer, he was told he would remember a person or experience that had caused an emotional blockage. He had to talk to the person, resolve the lingering problem and let it go.

Aaron was sceptical at first and insisted he wasn't going to invent problems or imagine people. But they popped up spontaneously. His mother and his father appeared, and there were other people and moments from his childhood that he had forgotten. An hour or two of unknotting the past left him sweating, weepy and exhausted, but cleansed.

The Journey therapist visited a couple more times once he was at home, but Aaron eventually decided he could take no more of this intense self-analysis. The night after the last session, he had a series of dreams. People hurried around as if in a hospital and individuals came briefly into focus. 'Hi, Aaron. How are you going? Are you doing well?' asked one woman before she rushed off, saying, 'Oh, Dave, Daveo – hold on a minute. Sorry, Aaron . . .' A man would seem to come in to remove a catheter from Aaron and apologise about the discomfort. 'You'll just have to put up with this for a moment.' He could see his mother sitting beside his bed, praying in the yellow light, and he knew it was the last minute of his life. In the dream, he felt himself let go and die.

This sequence repeated night after night: Hi, Aaron . . . Daveo . . . hold on a minute . . . put up with this . . . mother's prayer . . . death. Aaron was unnerved but he thought his nightmare was probably the result of stirring up old memories.

He had three days' radiotherapy on his hip and made plans to visit Gail in Brisbane before the next round of treatment. He woke one morning to find his left leg didn't work. It was floppy and disobedient and twitched as though the messages from his brain were being interrupted at his hip. Charlie gave him the okay to fly and Aaron staggered onto the plane. His leg jumped around under his tray table and the figures from his dreams appeared in his left field of vision. They were so real that he recognised them easily. He walked off the plane but while he waited for his luggage at the carousel, his leg began to dance uncontrollably, and Gail had to find an airport attendant and a wheelchair.

They drove home and Aaron went straight to bed. When he woke, it was dusk and the house was quiet. As he rose, the twitching in his leg rippled up through his body and turned into a single strong pulse that took control. An inner voice told him that if he didn't call out for help, he was going to die.

'MUM!' Although he yelled at the top of his voice, he couldn't hear himself. The last thing he remembered was falling towards the bed.

Gail heard his cry from the kitchen. She ran into the bedroom and found Aaron collapsed and rigid with his eyes rolled back and a seizure charging his body every few seconds. Cold fear filled the minutes between her emergency call and the arrival of an ambulance.

After a night of sedation, Aaron woke up in intensive care sporting a central line into his chest, an intravenous drip, an oxygen mask and a catheter. It was a depressingly familiar set-up. As he lay wondering what had happened to the missing hours, a nurse hurried in and smiled at him. 'Hello. How are you going?' Suddenly she was distracted and called to someone outside, 'Oh, Dave, Daveo . . . hold on a minute. Sorry, Aaron . . .' Then she disappeared. Aaron was stunned – it was the exact moment from his dream. What was going on?

There were also more fundamental questions to worry about. He was weakened by the storm that had raged through his body and didn't know if he would be able to stand up or walk or play the piano. Yet, there was a soothing calm to being wrung out and in a hospital bed surrounded by other patients. Gail returned during the morning with a smile that looked to Aaron as if it had been sent by angels. She was grateful to find her son alive.

All day he had a sense of déjà vu, but in this case the memories had occurred before the events. They were more like premonitions. A doctor came to his bed.

'We're going to take this catheter out. You'll just have to put up with this for a moment.'

'Don't I know you?' he asked another doctor. He recognised

a nurse and finished her sentence. At the same time, he had trouble forming his own.

Aaron was placed under close observation for further seizures. By the next day, he was still confined to bed and emotionally lower than he could remember ever feeling before. Between the constant interruptions, his mind kept repeating an old family video. He wasn't just reminiscing, however, because some of the scenes were unknown. Five-year-old Amy ran into the living room with her pink ballet tutu and wand. His stepfather, Giles, leaned over a telephone answering machine and recorded a message that made them all laugh. Everyone was ten or fifteen years younger and his mother had her daggy 1980s hairstyle. Aaron couldn't turn the tape off and even though they were happy memories, they seemed to be carrying him to an unavoidable conclusion.

That night, Gail slipped into his room and pulled up a chair beside his bed.

'I'm just going to sit here and pray,' she said.

Aaron's eyes shot open. No! There was his mother with the yellow light behind her. She hadn't settled into the position that was etched into his mind from the dream but it seemed inevitable. Aaron looked up at her face as she closed her eyes. That was it: the scene was set. He was going to die tonight. He had to disrupt the sequence.

'Mum,' he said, 'I really think I'll be okay tonight. You can go home.'

'I'll just sit here and do some quiet thinking,' she said.

He couldn't look at her. 'No, please, go home and get some sleep. Go!'

Aaron was shaken and tearful. Sleep was a long way off. The ward was dark but light seeped in from the corridor. In his drugged and dreamy state, he saw with unusual clarity the speckles of light and colour that play in the darkness behind closed eyelids.

An inner voice urged him, 'Look ahead, and see what you can see.' Nothing made sense but the outside world appeared to drift away. Aaron seemed to be staring into the far distance, yet all he could see were the dots in front of his closed eyes. Mentally he zoomed in and the dots became an intricate, tessellated pattern. It was a peaceful, mindless distraction from a desperate night. He was floating down to a void and one of the tessellations came into focus like a green mosaic tile. He let himself fall and smashed through the green wall. Now he was flying as if in a helicopter and knew where he was: it was the green computer grid that had appeared soon after his surgery, when his mind felt as though it was repairing and rebooting.

Way below him, Aaron could see a rolling sphere with perpendicular rows of green building blocks extending infinitely beyond the curved horizon. It looked like a giant information structure. As he swooped down, the blocks turned into more detailed columns and towers, and a vivid landscape burst into view with people running and flames burning along a grid of streets.

Beautiful symphonic music carried him forward and he lost contact with his body. He couldn't have told himself, 'Move your right arm' or 'Shake your left leg.' He knew he was in hospital, but he felt lost in the scene and didn't know how to get back. Perhaps he was on a dying journey, and yet he was compelled to go forward. He realised later that his eyes had peeled open and he was watching another dimension superimposed on the half-lit hospital room. People were walking along a road that was also the tray table, past a line of trees that was the curtains and a rickety fence that was the edge of his bed. With a great effort, he kicked his foot under the hill of bedclothes and, bang, the physical world came back into focus.

A nurse was asking, 'Are you okay, darling?'

The other world was not far away, though. It was as if he had stepped out of his body and seen more than he was supposed to see; he had visited an actual moment in some other place and time, just like the doctors and nurses who had played out their scenes in his dreams and then appeared in real time. Aaron wanted to go back there.

He rolled onto his side, facing the door and the corridor. He closed his eyes and travelled through the tessellations and down, down, until he reached a single square. He knew this time that when he opened his eyes, the ordinary setting in front of him would fit into another, extraordinary one. But what?

A medieval tableau opened up. On a cobblestone street, the night-lit windows of an inn showed people washing dishes while others sat talking at tables. Aaron was watching from a shed with knives and tools dangling from the ceiling. He could hear people talking and doors slamming. He thought, 'I'm actually here.' A few figures stumbled out the front door of the inn, one fell over and another gave him a playful kick. At the same time, Aaron was aware of a nurse walking towards him across the hospital ward and she paused to step around the little group.

That was enough. Aaron snapped himself out of his vision. Although he was still weak and unsteady on his legs, he got up and went out into the bright corridor. He sat down, rested his weary head in his hands and sobbed. Fascinated and frightened, he wondered again if he had been dying as he mentally left the ward and travelled to a place from which he might not return.

With little else to do, he became addicted to his time travels and, over the next four days, took off at least a dozen times. Only one other journey left a strong impression. Lying in bed wondering where he would go, he looked up into the bare corner of his room and found himself in a blue marble palace with massive columns along one wall. The grand hall was empty except for Aaron, who stood twenty metres from where the king might sit. He was in a temple dedicated to the gods.

When he talked to one of the nurses about what he had seen, she smiled. 'Those drugs are pretty cool, aren't they?'

No matter what drugs he was on, he didn't think his brain could invent all the places he had seen. Gail was open to the idea that he had entered another dimension and interpreted the trauma of his seizure and inner journeys as a necessary rebirth. He told her everything about his dreams and visions except for the scene in which he'd felt himself die while she prayed. When he confided that experience months later, she wept, believing she could have lost him.

His out-of-body travels were probably just hallucinations, the effect of the seizures or the drugs. Shaun Watson believed there was a connection with his seizures but he had no explanation for Aaron's particular visions. Most commonly, he said, people did not see familiar faces or figures, and most visions were static rather than active. But no two cases were the same. He had recently treated an elderly woman whose eyesight and brain function were deteriorating because of multiple sclerosis. At first everything she looked at was cracked or bubbled. Then she started seeing her late husband and other dead relatives. She knew they were hallucinations but, as they became more intrusive, she could smell and touch them and believed they were in the room with her. Steroids and anti-psychotic drugs eventually dispelled the visitors and calmed her mind.

Watson was more concerned about the *status epilepticus* that had sent Aaron to hospital – a continuous seizure that lasted forty-five minutes, causing stiffness, shaking and unconsciousness. That was a major medical emergency. However, Aaron had responded well to treatment and with a new medication, Dilantin, he had not relapsed. His new tumours were, of course, a serious problem, but appeared unrelated to the seizure.

'In the overall scheme of things, it's a relatively minor complication of successful surgery,' Watson concluded.

Whatever the doctors had to say, Aaron was profoundly changed by his latest trauma. Everything was different from the first time he had become ill. That had been brief and dramatic and ended triumphantly. This new episode kept taking unexpected twists and no one was offering a cure.

24

CLIMB EVERY MOUNTAIN

'I don't think I'm the man for you,' Charlie said, sitting at his desk dressed in blue cotton theatre pants and new high-tech hiking boots. He chewed an M&M while listening to a woman on the phone whose husband had been advised elsewhere against undergoing surgery on his tumour.

Charlie stood up and strode around the small room, bending his knees and testing his boots as if at any moment he might spring out the door. It was 30 June 2004. Fourteen-year-old Matthew Fiddick had died in January, his bravery and Charlie's persistence overtaken by increasingly aggressive tumours. From Charlie's perspective, it was a 'good death'. 'There was no pain and we knew if we let it go on, he would die a terrible, painful death.'

Such pragmatism was to be expected from a man who watched patients die every week, but it was hard to share. I wondered if he could say anything encouraging about Aaron's condition.

'As a scientist it shouldn't come as a shock,' he said. 'All you've

got to do is read the textbooks and they'll tell you that heman-
giopericytomas are malignant tumours with a high recurrence
rate. So, why it came as a shock, I think, is that I'd socialised
with Aaron a bit after the operation and his positive attitude
had rubbed off on me, and hopefully mine had rubbed off
on him, and we were both egging each other on, convincing
each other.

'I thought if the tumour came back it would come back in the
head. If you look at the literature, there are cases where it hasn't
recurred in the head but it's been throughout the body, in the
bone. The first thought was, oh my God, I should have given him
radiotherapy. But the literature says that giving radiotherapy at
the primary site decreases the recurrence rate at the primary site
but it doesn't decrease the incidence of bony metastases – the
principle being that the thing has metastasised before you even
attack the primary.'

So, the bomb had silently detonated. The neurosurgeon, with
all his years of training and the latest equipment, was powerless.
From now on, it seemed that Charlie could only watch while
others led the fight. If he sounded detached it was because, like
all doctors who faced death every day, he had to avoid sinking
into feelings of futility so he could keep going forward. It was
also because his patient continued to baffle and amaze him.

Aaron had left hospital and in April appeared at the big annual
fundraiser for the Cure for Life Foundation. He had helped
shape the ball into a comedy night called Laugh for Life –
featuring comedians such as Jackie Loeb, Peter Berner and Elliot
Goblet, and music from John Paul Young's Allstars and the young
boys of Indicator – so it was all the more disturbing for the guests
when he took the stage to report the downturn in his health. In
his tuxedo, he looked handsome but drained.

Charlie was pleased that seven neurosurgeons attended. His passion for the foundation sometimes wavered because politics was forcing the board to disperse its funds widely while his pet projects languished. Still, by mid-2004 he had been voted best teacher by the student doctors at Prince of Wales and, even without a steady flow of referrals within Australia, his practice was growing due to word of mouth and media attention. He was doing more surgery and lecturing overseas, especially in America.

'Have scalpel, will travel,' he said happily.

He had been appointed to the executive board of the International Society for Paediatric Neurosurgery. As his reputation for tackling difficult tumours continued to spread, more and more foreign patients were also coming to him. In one recent week, he had operated on children from the United States, South Africa and Indonesia, and in the last week of June, he had removed no fewer than sixteen brain tumours. The Centre for Minimally Invasive Neurosurgery was becoming truly international.

With success came restlessness; Charlie called it a midlife crisis. Over several years he had run a marathon, swum a long-distance ocean race and paddled a kayak marathon. For more than a decade, his children and career had been demanding enough; now that he had reached a comfortable plateau, he was looking for trouble again. By June, he was preparing to climb the two highest mountains in Ecuador. At 6267 metres and 5896 metres, the ice-capped Chimborazo and Cotopaxi are volcanoes that poke through the clouds above the Andes.

He was breaking in his boots and in a few weeks, on 3 September, he would set out with a team that included Peter Nakaji, the American neurosurgeon and experienced mountaineer, and Mark Coughlan, a South African who was his current visiting fellow. They would use crampons, ice picks and ropes.

Charlie was nervous. Six hundred people began the Cotopaxi climb each year. A hundred made it all the way. Twenty had died trying.

'But I like that,' he said. 'You can get too comfortable in your zone and when you get too comfortable, you forget the big world out there presents challenges to a lot of people. I like the fact that it is challenging me and making me apprehensive, because surgery doesn't do that to me anymore.'

He had trouble seeing how alike he and Aaron were in some ways – their drive, their optimism, their ambition to help others – and wondered about Aaron's decision to invite *Australian Story* back into his life, his willingness to suffer on camera. Did he want fame at any cost? It was a question often asked about Charlie, too. Both of them argued that their attention-seeking served a grander cause.

'If anyone's going to beat this, Aaron is,' he said. 'He reminds me of the Monty Python character who has his arms cut off and then his legs and never gives up. "'Tis but a scratch . . . Just a flesh wound."'

Charlie shared that never-say-die attitude, whether he was confronting the diseases that afflicted his patients, the critics who tried to topple his career or the physical dangers he sought out himself. The patients he attracted tended to be the same.

At least one of them was still fighting from his grave. Neil McKenzie, the New Zealand GP, had died in May 2003 after four operations. McKenzie was unreservedly grateful for the improved quality of life he'd enjoyed until three months before his death. He had lodged a complaint against his original neuro-surgeon and radiation oncologist in New Zealand for failing to inform him of all possible treatment options. All the neuro-surgeon had offered, said McKenzie, were palliative radiotherapy and the depressing words that 'there was nothing he could do', 'no surgery would be of benefit' and 'nobody survives these things'.

New Zealand's Health and Disability Commissioner began an inquiry into the complaint a few weeks before McKenzie's death. His widow, Gail, was determined to see it through. A serene, independent woman who owned an employment agency, she was worn down by having to relive her husband's illness but, in April 2004, she was vindicated. The Commissioner found that the neurosurgeon, though not the oncologist, had breached the ten-year-old Code of Health and Disability Services Consumers' Rights.

Ordered to apologise to Gail and to review his explanation of treatment options to future patients, the neurosurgeon wrote a letter that McKenzie's widow considered dutiful rather than sincere. In reiterating that glioblastomas were irremovable, he had missed the point. Sure enough, three months later he asked the Commissioner to take the unusual step of reopening his investigation.

Letters from several neurosurgeons in New Zealand and Australia backed their colleague. Others argued that surgical resection of such a tumour was an accepted practice and the neurosurgeon was obliged to present it as a real option. The Commissioner reached his decision quickly. In August 2004, he found that the neurosurgeon and those defending him had misconstrued his original opinion. The only test was what a reasonable patient would expect to be told. The appeal had failed and the investigation was closed.

Although Australia has no equivalent of New Zealand's Code of Health, the McKenzies' win was an important signal. It was, indirectly, a victory for Charlie over all the doctors who had neglected to tell their patients about his style of radical treatment or, worse, had warned them against him and turned their backs on those who sought his help.

When Charlie arrived home from Ecuador in the last week of September, there was plenty to celebrate. He had let his hair grow beyond its usual buzz cut as protection from the weather at the top of the world and a few flecks of grey showed in the dark sheen. He had survived his climb, even if he had not quite made the intended conquest.

On the final ascent to Cotopaxi, an icy peak despite being an active volcano, he had felt the hard numbness of frostbite in his fingers and the first signs of confusion from the thinning air. Every few minutes, he touched his nose and recited his Visa card number to make sure he hadn't lost his memory. At one point, his leg plunged through the snow into a crevasse and, when he looked down, all he could see was endless blackness below him. His only means of escape was to pull his leg up and leap over the void. He was exhausted, panting with every step, and on his hands and knees by the end. His mind was full of Genevieve and his daughters.

Charlie knew his self-imposed ordeal didn't compare with the suffering borne daily by his patients, but it gave him some insight. Sitting at his old wooden dining table on a warm spring evening with rain falling on the veranda, he said, 'It was so much like neurosurgery. You see a huge tumour and you think, "How am I going to remove that?" But you do it little bit by little bit, one step at a time, take a breath. And you get there.'

Soon after his return, he took a call from one of his medical soul mates. Fred Epstein was a leading American paediatric neurosurgeon who had established the Institute for Neurology and Neurosurgery at Beth Israel Hospital in New York City.

He described himself as 'the paediatric neurosurgeon of lost causes' and, like Charlie, argued, 'It's not a doctor's job to deprive a patient or a family of hope.'

Among his achievements was proving over the past twenty years, with new technology, that it was possible to remove low-grade, well-defined tumours from a child's fragile spinal cord and brain stem – a structure the thickness of a thumb that controls breathing, blood pressure, speech, swallowing, eye movement and other vital motor functions. Following his example, Charlie had removed many brain stem tumours in America and was getting the same good results in Sydney. The only obstacle was the Children's Hospital, where referrals were still scarce.

From his own experience, Epstein had warned Charlie that he would need five years to gain acceptance in Australia and that people would try to pull him down. He'd been proved right again. Now, fate reconnected the two men. In 2001, Epstein had been thrown off his bicycle and landed on his head, causing his brain to hit the back of his skull and tear a blood vessel. His helmet saved his life but he was in a coma for twenty-six days and, even after a long rehabilitation, knew he would not regain his skills as a surgeon and director of his state-of-the-art centre. By 2004, the institute was on a financial slide and Beth Israel agreed to sell it to the neighbouring St Luke's-Roosevelt Hospital. Ads were placed for a new head of paediatric neurology, and a senior specialist at the two hospitals who knew Charlie from Arkansas asked him to apply.

Charlie said no. He had put in five hard years at Prince of Wales and was reluctant to leave his Centre for Minimally Invasive Neurosurgery. He didn't want to return to the seven-days-a-week, publish-or-perish intensity of American work. There had been other offers and sometimes temptation pricked him. But when he picked his daughters up from school on Friday afternoons, his 'academic' day off from clinical work, he knew he was in the right place.

25

AN AUSTRALIAN STORY

Aaron was climbing mountains of his own throughout 2004. After the crises of the early part of the year, he had gone on to experience an astonishing sense of freshness and freedom. He knew it was probably due to physical reasons, even a chemically induced condition from his drugged stay in hospital, but he liked it all the same. While he generally saw himself as a tiny working part of the conglomeration of human beings on earth, in his newborn state he felt as if he were standing barefoot on the grass and wiggling his toes.

That feeling would fade but it left him more interested in daily achievements than ten-year plans, and more aware of his body's needs. Once again, he intended to immerse himself in music, and to work out the geometry and mathematics of the sounds he wanted to create. Stress had played a part in his breakdown, he was sure, and pure music – without the pressures of perform-ance and deadlines and finance – was his playground. ·

The world and his well-wishers would not be entirely shut out, though. While he was in hospital, a counsellor visited from the Quest for Life and told Aaron he already had the tools – control, challenge, commitment and connection – for beating his cancer. Quest for Life was started by Petrea King, who had been diagnosed with acute myeloid leukaemia as a young woman in 1983, and, since her recovery, had shared her knowledge of natural health and spiritual growth with many others suffering from life-threatening diseases. Aaron's old school sent him to a residential program run by Ian Gawler, a former vet who had famously cured himself of bone cancer with a combination of medicine, meditation, positive thinking and diet. Aaron liked the principles but after a couple of days fled the centre. His desperate, dying companions freaked him out. He wasn't one of them.

His mother found a nutritionist who claimed that if he followed her diet precisely for three months he would obliterate all signs of cancer. She swore that none of her patients had ever died. So, his days were awash with fresh juices and rich with vitamins, meditation and rest. There were also periodical visits to Prince of Wales for radiation as new spots appeared in his bones. With the largest tumours in his neck and rib shrunken to insignificance, Aaron felt stronger and defiant.

'I don't see how bone cancer can kill you. It's not like it's in a vital organ,' he told me one day. 'Twas but a scratch.

After being incapacitated for months, he was eager to get back to the piano. A chance meeting with a concert promoter, Andrew McKinnon, led to an invitation to perform again at the Opera House in October, this time with financial backing. How could he refuse? Once more, all resolutions to live a calm, introspective life were swept aside as he and Andrew debated whether he should play more solo classics, a symphonic program with orchestra or an all-Australian repertoire. The last would be the riskiest choice but it would also be a novelty for the Opera House and would fulfil his wish to support Australian composers.

In his usual methodical way, Aaron planned his program by visiting the Australian Music Centre's library of compositions and recordings every day for two weeks. He listened to the first minute of five hundred musical works, discarding those that didn't hook him immediately. He had to prove to the many doubters that Australian music could be as pleasing as the European masterpieces. Even he found a lot of what he heard dissonant and chaotic, as if it were written for personal catharsis and the fashions of the mid-twentieth century. It wouldn't be easy to draw a full Concert Hall audience and, as time hurried by, McKinnon faltered, suggesting they do a more conventional program incorporating a short tribute to Australian music. But Aaron had found sixteen pieces he was sure would make an exciting program. To his ear, each was written with a clarity of form, a mellifluous sound and a desire to communicate with listeners.

The decision was finalised when the Governor of New South Wales, Marie Bashir, invited Aaron to afternoon tea at Government House. As the music-loving patron of the Cure for Life Foundation, she had got to know Aaron well and had taken a keen interest in his health and his career. When he outlined the program of the Australian concert, she leaped out of her seat with an idea. That year, 2004, was the bicentenary of the suggestion by the English explorer Matthew Flinders that New Holland should be renamed Australia. Aaron's concert was the ideal way to celebrate.

In interviews, he was candid but optimistic about his health. A month after having radiotherapy on a painful lump in his rib, he wrote in a letter to his supporters:

Currently my bone cancer is stable and isn't spreading. I've recovered well from radiation treatment and as long as I keep fighting it, I won't need any more treatment for now. I'm finally looking forward to putting the difficulties behind me and getting on with things!

On Friday 8 October, the Governor introduced him to an audience of almost a thousand people. The evening challenged them as it did Aaron, alone at the Australian-made Stuart piano and ranging through the history of Australian music. He began with the romantic Concert Study No. 3 in C sharp minor written in 1935 by Miriam Hyde, who at ninety-one was Australia's oldest living composer. Two hours later, he finished with Sonny Chua's 1989 *Dance, Dance, Dance*, described by the young composer as a celebration of movement, happiness and life. Peter Sculthorpe watched from a box as Aaron played his hauntingly lovely *Djilile*, which recalled an Aboriginal melody from Arnhem Land and the cry of a duck on a billabong.

As a business venture the night was a minor disaster, burning McKinnon and confirming that Australians were still largely indifferent to their country's serious music. But for Aaron, it represented a different kind of success. His body had held up under the duress of a long, athletic performance filmed by the ABC cameras for a planned second episode of *Australian Story*. And he had carried an audience along on his musical adventure.

After a few weeks' recovery, Aaron took his concert to Fremantle on the west coast, where the evening was a fundraiser for the Cure for Life Foundation organised by Anne Glaskin, mother of the little girl Lily, whose death had so upset Charlie's daughters.

As Aaron's hands ran up and down the keyboard, one wrist showed flashes of yellow. Graham Mackie, the promoter who had brought him over there, explained to the audience that a week earlier he had been at a West Australian tourist lookout and found a Dutch woman reading the concert flyer on the side of his car. After asking about Aaron's story, she showed Mackie a wide yellow rubber band on her wrist.

'Lance Armstrong gave this to me,' she said, 'and I'm going to put it on your wrist, and when you see Aaron, you must transfer it to his wrist.'

The band was inscribed with Armstrong's motto, *Live strong*. Aaron slid it over his hand and would never take it off.

26

BODY AND SOUL

It seemed a perfect coincidence to Aaron that on 16 August 2005, the fourth anniversary of his brain surgery, he should be sitting at a dining table in the smallest sail of the Sydney Opera House with a Catholic priest.

Father Joseph Carola, however, disagreed. 'There is no coincidence,' he said, with a firm shake of his head. 'It's providence, God providing.'

After a gourmet dinner at the restaurant Guillaume at Bennelong, the two men hurried to the Opera Theatre for the opening night performance of Mozart's *Don Giovanni*. They came close to missing the curtain as Father Carola was stopped by a security guard, who told him to leave his bulky shopping bag in the cloakroom. The plump, bespectacled man with black robes and an American accent would have made an unlikely terrorist. But who could be sure in these nervous times, just five weeks after suicide bombers had attacked the London Underground?

It was a light-hearted evening for the pianist and the priest, but much more than a casual outing. An unbreakable bond had formed between Aaron and Father Carola during their four meetings. This was to be the last before the Jesuit priest returned to Rome.

'Now I know why I was sent to Australia,' he told Aaron.

Father Joseph Carola had come reluctantly. Raised in Boston and trained by the Jesuits in America as a high school language teacher, he had followed a vocation to educate other young priests and help rebuild the struggling clergy at its heart, in Rome. Having earned his doctorate, he taught theology to a cosmopolitan student body at the Pontifical Gregorian University founded by Saint Ignatius Loyola in 1555, two blocks from the Trevi Fountain and a brisk walk from the Vatican. He had sung several times at masses celebrated by Pope John Paul II and had had audiences with the Polish pontiff.

When it came to the last stage of spiritual formation before taking his final vows – a seven-month period of study and prayer spent overseas – he had asked to be sent to Slovakia, where he admired the Jesuits for their endurance of prison and hard labour under the Communist regime. But God and his father superior demanded otherwise: Australia would fit the requirement that he do his tertianship in an English-speaking country. When providence brought him to Sydney in January 2005, he feared he would find a less traditional Catholicism and an earthbound, secular society.

Installed with the other foreign Jesuits at Canisius College in the northern Sydney suburb of Pymble, he began to relax. In April, he was sent to Brisbane to guide a group of ordinary parishioners through three weeks of spiritual exercises. Among them was Gail Puckett, Aaron's mother.

Gail had already shown that in times of trouble she turned back to her Catholic roots. Her life had been unsettled for months now. She had given up her teaching job at the end of the previous year, thinking she would devote more time to her son. She hoped Aaron would move into the house she and Giles had recently built on a hill outside Brisbane. It was just like the house Aaron had dreamed about after his surgery. They talked of building a cabin in the garden where he could sleep and compose. But they both knew he would die of boredom.

So, Gail was torn between her husband and children in Brisbane and her son in Sydney. She took up the education degree she had dropped years before and started going sporadically to the local Catholic church, mainly for the joy of singing in the choir. But with more time to think, worries crashed in: Aaron's cancer, Andrew's broken wrist, Amy's boyfriend troubles, and her father's latest illness all seemed to weigh on her equally. When she heard about a retreat at the church, she signed up, interested in the idea of meditation and discussion with a Jesuit priest.

Father Carola arrived with his own sorrow. After a long public illness, Pope John Paul II had finally died at 5.37 am on 3 April, Sydney time, as Carola noted in his diary. It was as though his own father had died and he could not go home to bury him. Watching the funeral on television, he wondered why he was on the other side of the world. The same question arose when Cardinal Ratzinger, whose masses he had attended and discussed with his students for five years, was elected Pope Benedict XVI on 19 April.

He worked out the answer: 'It was important for me to see how the rest of the world experiences the death of a pope and the election of a new pope, and how the rest of the world and I were dependent on the media.' He countered media images of Ratzinger as 'the Enforcer' by telling the Brisbane parish his own stories of the man's compassion.

Gail was inspired by Father Carola from their first meeting and a talk he gave debunking the popular novel *The Da Vinci Code*. During her retreat, they met twice a week to talk about prayer and passages of scripture. She confided her troubles and they seemed lighter when she left him. Before he returned to Sydney, she gave him some of Aaron's CDs and his phone number.

On a Saturday morning in May, Father Carola made the two-hour bus trip from Pymble to Bondi. Aaron met his visitor on the esplanade, and they ate breakfast and strolled above the white sand. Father Carola was impressed to find that Aaron really was the concert pianist his proud mother had described. He played the organ himself. At his aunt's place, Aaron insisted Father Carola sit down at the piano and play, which was a treat for the music-starved priest.

Once again, Aaron's plans for a quiet year of healing and composition had come unstuck. His contacts at the Sydney Opera House had offered him a date for another solo performance and, despite the financial and health risks, his imagination took off. By the time he met Father Carola, he had the Concert Hall booked for 17 September and had arranged a series of smaller performances as practice runs for the main event. After attending one at Cranbrook School, Father Carola said, 'The vital spirit that came through in his music was a glimpse into his soul, where God dwells. There's so much life that comes out through his music. There's that hidden cancer but the life outshines it completely.'

The new Pope had announced that his predecessor was worthy of sainthood and, rather than waiting the traditional five years after death, the process should begin immediately. There were two stages, beatification and canonisation, and for each, proof was needed that God had worked a miracle of healing through the candidate's intercession. Millions of Catholics began to direct their prayers through their late pontiff.

Father Carola thought, 'Pope John Paul II is a saint in heaven, there's no doubt about it. I know he will one day, probably in the not too distant future, be beatified then hopefully canonised. It's going to happen, God is going to perform a miracle through the intercession of Pope John Paul II, so why can't it be for someone like Aaron McMillan?'

Father Carola was already praying for a woman in England who had been stabbed and left paraplegic by a man who tried to kidnap her two-year-old son. His prayers for her, and for Aaron, were, above all, for their physical and spiritual healing. But if God could also use them for the cause of beatification, he would be overjoyed.

Aaron's phone rang incessantly with inquiries from concerned friends and even strangers, so the priest made a point of not calling. Busy with his spiritual duties, he was unaware of the physical drama that was about to test his prayers.

On 8 July 2005, eighteen months after his Brisbane seizure, Aaron went for a routine brain scan. He had no particular sense of foreboding, so it was a devastating shock to peep at the scans and see a small but definite shadow.

'Fuck,' he said, and strode out of the radiology department, his Aunt Dene trailing behind him. Aaron called Charlie, who was in surgery; he called back a few hours later. Aaron was lucky to catch him – just back from a neurosurgery meeting in Morocco, he was leaving in a few days to teach his regular endoscopy course in the United States, coming home via New Zealand.

They both remembered the insignificant dot on the previous scans. Now there was a growth several centimetres in diameter close to the site of his old tumour. But there were differences: this tumour was centred on the vein of Galen, that fragile confluence of all the major veins draining the deepest parts of the brain, whereas the original tumour had only touched its lower edge. Several smaller spots circled the main one like moons.

'What should I do about the concert?' asked Aaron.

It was an echo of the attitude that had annoyed Charlie when they first met, the concern for getting on with his career when survival was more urgent. But this time, Charlie encouraged him.

'Do the things you most want to do,' he replied. 'Pretend you've got six months to live. Would you look back and say, "That was the best way to spend my time"?'

'Charlie! Don't say that.'

'It's not going to happen,' said Charlie. 'But just pretend.'

He really didn't think the brain tumour would kill Aaron. Its position around the vein of Galen was precarious. It sat against the parietal-occipital lobes, close to the mid-line of the brain but this time slightly to the left rather than the right. If it grew to a size that put pressure on the brain tissue, it could affect sensory input and cause problems with memory, left–right orientation, speech, writing – and reading and playing music. But Charlie judged that it was growing slowly and there were no symptoms yet. Surgery was a risk not worth taking. Besides, with new cancer spots popping up in Aaron's flesh and bones all the time, removing one would be like swatting a single fly amid a swarm.

Unable to act, Charlie retreated into the relativities of his profession. He had just seen a forty-year-old man, the father of young children, whose low-grade tumour he had removed a year earlier. Now it had turned malignant. According to the literature, that very rarely happened. On the other hand, he would operate on Sunday, before his flight, on a man with an anaplastic tumour declared inoperable by his doctors in South Africa. Charlie believed he could buy him four or five good years. That was success.

'I can't help thinking of all the people who die within a year of their diagnosis,' Charlie told me. 'Aaron has lived five times longer than most people with a malignant brain tumour.'

For Aaron, Charlie's 'six months' sounded like a death sentence, the way 'six weeks' had at their first encounter. To head off despair, he did his usual meditation, focusing on his cancers and mentally dissolving them. His concert would go ahead. 'I want to find elegant ways through everything without crashing and burning. Cancelling the Opera House would mean cancelling everything,' he said. 'I know I can beat the cancer.'

His deep meditations over the weekend seemed to have reduced the lumps he could feel in his bones. A swelling in his arm had almost disappeared. A painful spot at the base of his spine made it hard to practise but he was certain it would get better. There was still an appointment with Bob Smee to endure.

Aaron blamed neither of his doctors for his suffering, though he sometimes found Charlie's brisk advice cavalier and Smee's bluntness depressing. But he reasoned, 'Charlie's supporting me a hundred per cent. He sees hundreds of people dying every year. So, I can't nitpick. Never has it been the case where they missed something on a scan. Both of them had access to all the scans and I've cross-checked. I'm not disappointed by them; I'm disappointed by my situation.'

I accompanied Aaron to Smee's office, where he explained the appearance of his new brain tumour and Charlie's decision to watch its development for three or four months before considering surgery. Smee looked at the scans: there was a pale lump measuring about four by three centimetres near the wide delta of the vein of Galen, and four more tiny spots. But Aaron picked up on a piece of good news. The scan showed no big lumps at the top of his neck where the cancer had begun.

'Dr Teo believes I can fight the cancer on my own terms with diet and meditation and that in three months it might be smaller or the same,' he said, putting his own spin on Charlie's opinion.

Smee's reaction was patient but clear. 'I'm not overly impressed with just leaving it for three or four months. We have to guesstimate the growth rate prior to this . . .'

'The fact that this one is the size of a grape compared to a tennis ball last time–'

'It's more than a grape,' Smee said.

'Well, a grape and a half . . . I have no symptoms, so there's no reason I'd say I should have radiotherapy. It's not easy at all to know which way to go . . . I hate being in this position. I didn't plan this four years ago.'

'No one plans to be in this position. You face the dilemma many patients have of seeing two specialists and getting contrary views.' Smee explained that a bigger lump would be harder to treat because it came in contact with more healthy brain tissue, which was vulnerable to radiation. Even now, radiation could cause Aaron to lose power in his hands. The question was whether he could still have radiotherapy if he wanted it later.

'It's never untreatable,' said Smee. 'I treat people's whole head with success – it depends on their circumstances and what you mean by success. There are no rights or wrongs.'

'I believe I can overcome it myself,' Aaron said.

'Tremendous. Go for it.'

Aaron grinned as he stood up to go. 'I'll get back to it.'

Smee told me after Aaron had left the room, 'I think he should be treated. The problem is that Aaron has a significant amount of faith in surgery, and radiotherapy can make surgery harder. That weighs heavily on him . . . The aim is to give him as much good-quality life as possible. We tinker round the edges. Do I think he's going to be alive in five years? Aaron asked me that when we first met and I said no. That hasn't changed.'

The doctor looked weary rather than sad as he called his next patient.

27

THE POPE'S MIRACLE

Towards the end of July 2005, Aaron spent a week at his grandparents' house on the NSW Central Coast. He had taken the paperwork for his concert but as the days went by in the hard, narrow bed and the overheated rooms, he was dizzy and ached in all his bones. After a few minutes at the piano, the pain became unbearable. His brain tumour had also begun to hurt since he found out about it. He tried sleeping in a chair and standing against a wall, but the only relief came from lying weightlessly in a hot bath. He needed help.

It seemed only minutes after he had dragged himself up the steps to the Bondi flat that Father Carola was on the phone, hearing the latest bad news and suggesting another visit. So many people had prayed for Aaron that he hadn't put much emphasis on the priest's offering. But he liked the man and his kindness and agreed to meet him.

On his way to mass at St Mary's Cathedral in the city on

Sunday 7 August, Father Carola bought smoked salmon and chicken for lunch. Inside the stone cathedral, he offered mass for Aaron. Then he caught the bus to Bondi and spread his feast out on the kitchen table. The two men ate, talked about their spiritual lives, played the piano and watched videos of Aaron's *Australian Story* appearance and his birthday party on the boat.

It was time for Father Carola to leave and begin a week's silent retreat. As he said goodbye, though, some deeper instinct took hold of him and dispelled his habitual shyness. He wanted to pray over Aaron. It was not Father Carola's usual way and he didn't want to make Aaron uncomfortable, but he knew God had given him this opportunity. He grabbed Aaron by the arm.

'Come here, one second. Sit down,' he said, guiding Aaron onto a kitchen chair. 'I want to pray over you and pray for your healing.'

Father Carola sat and placed his right hand on Aaron's head and his left hand on his shoulder. With the sound of the surf rushing at the rocks outside, he prayed aloud, asking the Father to send a spirit of healing upon Aaron, the spirit by which Jesus healed. He addressed Mary, who cares for children and draws her Son's attention to those in particular need. He prayed through the intercession of Pope John Paul II for God to heal Aaron both physically and spiritually. And, if it should be God's will, for this to be one of the miraculous, revelatory moments which led to the beatification of one of His servants. He finished by tracing the sign of the cross with his thumb on Aaron's forehead. The Pope had done the same for Father Carola on 21 June 1993, when the young priest had attended his mass.

Aaron lay awake with pain that night. Next morning, however, he got out of bed with ease. He listened to a Mozart piano concerto and leaned against a wall in the hallway while his bath filled. A weary peace flowed through him. It was like the end of a long journey, as if someone had lifted a hitchhiker's pack from his back and he finally realised how tired he was.

Even greater changes became noticeable during the day. The largest cancers, which had created distinct swellings on his rib and upper arm, had shrunk to almost nothing. He could walk and sit and stand with a freedom he hadn't experienced for weeks. He cried tears of relief and astonishment. How could cancer exist in the pure peace he felt?

Before the day was over, Aaron called on his downstairs neighbour, Roselle Gowan, and pieced together the last twenty-four hours. Roselle, a lively Irish woman who had moved into the building with her husband the previous year, was the only person who had touched the tender lumps on Aaron's body and remembered clearly how the 'orange' in the flesh of his upper arm had felt. Pressing her fingers on those spots now, she could barely feel them.

When Aaron phoned and left a message on Father Carola's voicemail, the priest was still on retreat. 'Joseph, this is Aaron McMillan here,' he said. 'It's so hard to express this in a phone message. But I wanted to tell you that the next morning after you visited me, when I woke up, there was a profound difference in the size of the lumps on my bones, on my body, and I attribute that to your visit and your prayer. And I was very, very humbled and I cried, and I thanked you and I thanked the prayer you had said because something really profound happened . . .'

Aaron's night with Father Carola at the Opera House on 16 August floated on a sense of wonderment mixed with the sensuality of food, wine and music. The priest had emerged from his silence that morning. Aaron wanted to be clear about the fact that he was a religious innocent, no more than 'a sort of sort of

Catholic', and that this experience, while significant, was not a road-to-Damascus conversion.

'I feel more human than Christian,' he explained. 'I've always tried to not be too religious but rather to set an example, as religion teaches you, to be a good person, to love thy neighbour, help others, be selfless.' As they ate dessert, he pointed out that he had been baptised as a Catholic but never made his first communion. 'I hope you're not disappointed,' he said with an apologetic frown.

Father Carola stopped spooning his ice-cream and smiled. 'I'm not disappointed. It gives me something to look forward to.'

Several days later, I drove through the rain to Pymble, to visit the priest at Canisius College, a cluster of sober brick buildings among flowering English gardens. He was packing his few belongings for his return to Rome. We sat in armchairs in a small, sparse room while he explained warmly, but with old-fashioned formality, how important his meeting with Aaron had been, especially for himself. He had been most struck by the tears Aaron shed after their shared prayer. They were not tears of sorrow or self-pity or frustration.

'They're the tears that only God can give and they come from an overwhelming experience of consolation when God suddenly takes us by the hand. You shed those tears of joy in the most un-expected way and it's all-encompassing. When the Lord works in this way, He does so in order to reassure us of his profound love, and it's so precious. I'm greatly humbled to be able to witness God's love in a way you can touch.'

I wondered whether he was aware, while offering sincere belief in a healing, that Aaron might be devastated if no miracle occurred. The question didn't trouble Father Carola. In his view, Aaron had found deep peace for the first time in four years and that was no false hope. It was a huge reality.

'With the setting of the sun each day, all the living are one day closer to death, not just him. What I can be absolutely assured of is that God will provide for Aaron and that He will never abandon him. That doesn't necessarily mean that he'll be healed physically, but the Lord will bring great good. If Aaron one day were to die in great peace and joy and overwhelmed by the love that God has for him, I would wish that for everybody.' He paused. 'Not that I'd be disappointed if it was delayed in Aaron's case by a few decades. Do I believe God has worked a miracle for Aaron McMillan? Yes. Has it resulted in some physical healing? Yes. Will it result in a complete healing? That remains to be seen, but I hope and pray that it will. Every day of my life I will pray for him.'

A few days after our meeting, the priest left Sydney bound for Rome. On his last night at Canisius College, he sat in his small room until two o'clock in the morning writing a letter to Aaron. In page after page of perfect, tiny handwriting, he went over the events and revelations of the past weeks, quoting the Bible and repeating his promise of prayer. He described Aaron's music and his heroic struggle with cancer as his joint vocations and his ways of inspiring millions of people. And he laid out his hope that the 'drinking water' of Aaron's natural goodness would be transformed through the Eucharist, or Holy Communion, into the fine wine of God's love.

The letter was waiting when Aaron and Roselle arrived home from a weekend at Peter Crisp's country property, where Aaron had given another concert in the corrugated-iron gallery. The euphoria of the previous week was, for the moment, overwhelmed by fatigue and pain. Trying to decipher Father Carola's monkish script made Aaron's head ache. He took the letter downstairs and closed his eyes while Roselle read it aloud to him in her dancing Irish accent. She watched the tension leave his face as the pure message flowed over him again.

'Aaron,' she said when she reached the end, 'it's like a love letter from God.'

28

A DANGEROUS GAME

At twelve years old, Aaron had become engrossed in a book about the lives of the great composers. One day at his grandparents' house, he was reading while his grandmother cooked dinner, and the more he read, the more alarmed he became by how many composers had died young.

'Hey, Nan,' he said, speaking to her over the kitchen bench. 'Did you know that Schubert died when he was thirty-one and Mozart died when he was thirty-five and Chopin died when he was thirty-nine?'

Marjorie turned from the stove and looked seriously at her ambitious, golden-haired grandson. 'Aaron, I worry about you,' she said. 'It's a dangerous game, that composing.'

As an adult he recounted the story to illustrate his grandmother's sweet naivety. 'My grandmother never tells jokes but everything she says is funny,' he told the audience at one of his concerts. At twenty-eight, however, he was of the age when many of his heroes were reaching their peak and some were nearing their end. Though he wouldn't have put it so bluntly, he was still contemplating his composing career while he stared death in the face. Even now, he was too restless and too much in need of an income to sit alone and write.

Buoyed by his encounters with Father Carola, he got on with preparing his third solo concert at the Sydney Opera House. He had the idea of a program of works written by the great composers when they were young. Some were only beginning to compose, and others, such as Bach and Tchaikovsky, would write most of their solo keyboard pieces later. But it was an extraordinary creative output by young men, and the music expressed a clear energy and exuberance. Beethoven wrote his famous *Pathétique Sonata* at twenty-eight; Schumann wrote *Carnaval* at twenty-four; Chopin was a tubercular twenty-eight when he wrote his Nocturne in D flat, and only twenty-one when wrote the first of his Ballades.

In the lead-up to the concert on 17 September, Aaron tested himself at a series of recitals. The most important of these was scheduled for Saturday 27 August at Glenaeon Rudolf Steiner School, which was establishing a music scholarship in his name. His great supporter, the Governor of New South Wales, would launch the scholarship and he would play.

On the morning of the recital, Aaron sneezed. Pain ricocheted into his rib and stayed there. Almost immobilised, he called on Roselle, who spent most of the day pleading with the local chemist to supply prescription painkillers without a prescription.

When Charlie's mobile rang, he was in a lab at Prince of Wales with fifteen neurosurgeons and six severed heads. He was winding up a successful three-day symposium on keyhole techniques and, as usual, neurosurgeons from the United States, Germany and

Japan had come to learn from him and share their experiences. This time he was also pleased to see a few of his Australian colleagues.

The doctors, all men, clustered in small groups around the heads, which were male as well but elderly, with shaved scalps, their eyes and mouths sealed, and deep lines etched in their pickled flesh. Their individuality was reduced to a hooked nose, a jowly chin, a scarred brow.

'Each time someone donates their body, they save a life,' said Charlie respectfully before each team started rolling a head around the table and drilling holes in its skull.

'The endoscope can be a deadly instrument if used the wrong way. I get called once a month to be an expert witness on one of these cases in the US. Make sure everything is perfect before you open the dura. It often takes an hour and a half to prepare and seven minutes to operate. It's a beautiful, bloodless operation if everything is right.'

The doctors prodded the thin metal casing of the endoscopes into the narrow passageways of the brain until they reached the deepest space, the third ventricle, hoping they hadn't poked or torn anything precious on the way. Fortunately, the old blokes who had donated their bodies wouldn't suffer. By early afternoon, their skulls were punctured like bowling balls.

Among the American visitors was Peter Nakaji. I wanted to know what he thought about Aaron's derailed success. 'Most of these tumours recur because they're cancer,' he said. 'Without surgery, Aaron would have died within a year. He's done quite well, even though you don't feel that when the end comes.'

Aaron could finally take the edge off his pain after Charlie authorised his drugs over the phone but he still felt as if he'd been shot in the chest. The tumour spot in his rib had been wrenched

241

by his sneeze and would take days to calm down. Knowing he would have difficulty performing a recital a few hours later, he had already contacted another pianist. Lukas Opacic, a rising star at sixteen, was preparing for his own recital at the Sydney Conservatorium in October and agreed to share the evening at Glenaeon.

The school hall was crammed with teachers, pupils and parents. Aaron's mother and grandparents and friends leaned forward in their seats as he walked onstage with as little extraneous movement as possible.

'Many of you are aware that I'm battling bone cancer, which has the ability to rise up and grab you . . .' he said, pushing out the words from his painful torso. He explained that his publicist, Philippa Drynan, had helped him find Lukas, and he introduced the younger pianist with a flourish of compliments.

At the piano, he set his jaw and performed his three pieces through excruciating pain. He had already accepted that he could not carry a night at the Opera House alone three weeks later, and had asked some of Australia's best young pianists to join him. Despite the short notice, they all leaped at the opportunity to help and to appear on Sydney's best stage. One of them was his old friend Tamara Anna Cislowska, the daughter of his teacher, Neta Maughan, and now an international performer. Another was Clemens Leske, just back from an appearance with the London Philharmonic. Then there was Evgeny Ukhanov, a brilliant Ukrainian musician who lived in Sydney. And now, having heard Lukas Opacic, Aaron invited him to join the group.

'It's not every day you get to play solo in front of a few thousand people at the Opera House,' said Aaron at home in an armchair the day after the Glenaeon concert, trying to recover quickly for the last weeks' frenzy of programming, ticketing, publicity and rehearsal. 'These pianists have performing opportunities but it's very hard. I know there are audiences out there for these musicians but ninety-five per cent of the whole challenge is to get the audiences – the performing is really just the icing on the cake. Otherwise, there are all these talented young musicians who don't have anyone to play for.

'This is a life-and-death turning point for me. I'm proud of the fact that despite all this rubbish I've had to deal with, I've still ticked every box; I've still managed to do things. This time yesterday the probability of me getting out of the house was remote and yet it all went well and everyone had a lovely time. Somehow I found a way to make things happen and to fulfil projects and promises . . . I'm just being asked to wait, stand in the corner and face the wall.'

Once he pulled off this concert at the Opera House, Aaron knew it would be time to stop performing, at least for a while.

'Maybe my body's interpreting this as stressful and there's a subconscious thing that is keeping the cancer hanging around. Consciously, I feel happy and I love putting on these events, but there always was that pull towards being truly creative, because performing is not truly creative. It's interpretive, like acting as opposed to writing. There must be something eating away at me for not fully getting into my creativity and learning the fundamentals of what music is and how it fits together. I've linked that move into giving myself a chance to get better and I think that's because composing gives you the freedom to take your time to think about bigger things than who's going to phone you about what next, and to step outside the bubble within which you've become unwell.

'It's hard to know why I've got cancer. It might just be a virus, a bug, parasites; there's so many ideas. To me, this concert is showing my appreciation to Charlie and accepting my position as having cancer and to help that cause, and then stepping out of that environment I've pretty much been in for ten years and really trying to make a complete break into a different type of living. It will be interesting to see how it pans out, because I have an absolute love of people. I'm not a hermit and I can't live in a composing shack by a lake and write symphonies until I drop dead writing my ninth. It's not me.'

29

THE SHOW GOES ON

Four days before the concert, Aaron sank into a fog of pain and medication. Roselle found him and roused him to do a radio interview. Then he slid away again. A series of scans revealed a large tumour in the fourth thoracic vertebra, T4, between his shoulderblades. Wrapped around the spinal cord, in a short time the tumour would have strangled the nerves and left him paraplegic. Emergency radiotherapy began the process of beating it back. By Wednesday morning, three days before the concert, Aaron was leaning against a hill of pillows in the hospital ward.

'My torso is the make or break,' he said. 'My arm bones are fine. My leg bones are fine. My finger bones are fine.'

On Friday, denial and determination had to give way to a decision. Was he really able to play? He took himself home to see his mother, sister and friends who had come down from Brisbane. Late at night, when they had all gone, he sat at the piano in his bedroom with Roselle at his side. Lifting his arms to the keyboard caused a searing pain in the centre of his back. Pressing the keys took more strength than he could find.

Six notes emerged . . . and then silence. His hands fell to his lap and he looked at Roselle.

'I'm sorry. I can't do it.'

On Saturday morning, he made a phone call from hospital to Alexander Gavrylyuk, another young Ukrainian pianist living in Sydney. At twenty-one, Alexander was becoming a star in Japan and Europe, and in April had won the prestigious Arthur Rubinstein International Piano Master Competition. With less than twelve hours' notice, he agreed to take Aaron's place in the concert.

By extraordinary coincidence, Erica Jacobsen, the piano-playing registrar who had cared for Aaron in 2001, had saved Alexander's life nine months later, after his head was smashed into a telegraph pole in a car accident. She and a plastic surgeon had to drag the compressed bone above his eye back into place without damaging the frontal lobe of his brain.

'The surgeons saved my life – with the help of God, of course,' Alexander told me. 'This accident gave me a lot of material for thinking and for understanding music better. I experienced some things not many people have seen and that is really important because music is about the deepest human feelings.'

Aaron discharged himself from hospital for the day and his first stop was Charlie's house. The evening's entertainment and a pre-concert dinner organised by Roselle were fundraisers for the Cure for Life Foundation. As long as he could stand, he would be there.

Charlie had flown in that morning from a conference in Vancouver. He had expected to miss the concert, but when word reached him that Aaron was struggling from hospital to be there, he caught the first flight home. He was surprised when Aaron dropped round for morning tea and a briefing on his health and the night's agenda. Still doing the right thing, even though he was thin and breathless, his handshake weak and his muscles wasted.

At Bondi, with help from his Brisbane friends and a dose of morphine, Aaron spent the afternoon printing two thousand revised programs before easing himself into his dinner suit. One of his mother's former pupils, eleven-year-old Benji Wilton, had become another of Aaron's protégés as they worked together to channel his hyperactivity into usefulness. Tonight the boy was responsible for carrying Aaron's morphine supply and carefully placed the two fat plastic syringes in his pocket.

In the restaurant where Aaron and Father Carola had dined a month earlier, a hundred Cure for Life supporters ate Guillaume Brahimi's fine food. They could barely imagine the will it took for Aaron to stand and address them.

'Just in the last few hours, Alexander Gavrylyuk has taken over from me, [and he is] one of the world's great young pianists . . . It's emotional, because it means I cannot perform myself, but I can give others an opportunity.'

For a few seconds, he couldn't speak. Emotion swelled his throat as he heard his own words. He felt with a thud the pain and disappointment of his loss. Yet, there was also pride in the musicians he was showcasing.

Charlie took over and tried to lift the mood. 'Aaron's cancer is a bit different from most, a very rare kind,' he said. 'People can live with it for years. Even with secondaries, Aaron still has this hope, which is not only in his heart but in the literature, that he will live to a ripe old age.' He spoke about the need for research into the most aggressive brain tumours, glioblastomas. Already he could see a far-off light. The foundation was funding a study that had identified genetic abnormalities associated with those tumours and the possibility that they were treatable.

'If we continue this way, we might find a cure.'

In the maze behind the Concert Hall stage, the five pianists were running through their pieces according to Aaron's roster. Wild eyes and blasts of music met Aaron, still wearing his hospital bracelet, as he opened each door. The ABC radio presenter Margaret Throsby was host for the night. Sitting with Aaron in his dressing room, she briskly absorbed the changes to the program and to his condition.

Aaron stilled himself with a few minutes' meditation, then asked Benji for the hit of morphine that would get him through the next two hours. Benji pulled the two syringes out of his pocket. Both were empty. The contents had leaked in a damp mess.

Aaron didn't panic. Out in the corridor, he fumbled with the syringes like an addict in a back lane. 'It's okay, it's okay,' he repeated, moaning and tilting his head back to swallow the last bitter drops from each syringe. He managed to extract about half a millilitre instead of the necessary five.

He settled onto a chair in the control room at the side of the stage, from where he would watch the concert through glass and hear it through speakers. Technicians moved back and forth across the panel of switches, manipulating lights, sound and performers.

Onstage, Margaret Throsby began. 'It's a remarkable battle, this battle that Aaron McMillan is waging. He's the Lance Armstrong of piano players, I think.'

Alexander Gavrylyuk strode out and sat at the Steinway that Aaron had broken in before his 2003 concert. An intense, compact figure with a grim scar on his forehead, he flung himself into 'Rondo alla Turca' from Mozart's Piano Sonata No. 11. Lukas Opacic played the Ballade No. 4 by Chopin, rushing slightly under the pressure of the night, and Evgeny Ukhanov ended the first half of the program with the exquisite Schumann *Carnaval* that Aaron had once hoped to play.

With his eyes closed, his head dulled and his torso electric with pain, Aaron heard the music as a distant serenade. At interval, he found Evgeny in the backstage corridors and put an arm on his shoulder. Evgeny expected him to be sad but Aaron expressed a woozy elation. He laughed as they passed a Viennese dandy, no doubt a cast member from *Don Giovanni*.

'I practised that piece so hard and it's wonderful to hear you playing for me,' he said. 'I feel like it's all that work and you are shining for everybody. It doesn't matter that I wasn't able to play.'

Tamara Anna Cislowska, her red hair offset by a deep blue skirt, launched into Liszt's *Dante Sonata*. She took the audience on a musical journey into purgatory before allowing them to reach paradise. Clemens Leske played serenely through Liszt's *Petrarch Sonnet No. 104* and Stravinsky's 'Shrove-tide Fair' from the ballet *Petroushka*. Then, for a moment's fun, he broke into 'Flight of the Bumblebee' by Rimsky-Korsakov, a short, manic arrangement by Georges Cziffra.

Alexander finished the program with Etude in D Minor by Scriabin, but when Margaret Throsby returned, she said, at Aaron's request, 'I think we could ask Alexander back for an encore, don't you?'

He had chosen another, wilder version of Mozart's 'Rondo

alla Turca' by a young Russian pianist, Arcadi Volodos. Intricate, fast and funny, Volodos's transcription struck Aaron as *Bugs Bunny* cartoon music and made him laugh.

Aaron made it through drinks in the green room. Around midnight, it was time to turn inwards, away from the crowd and the music. Benji's father drove him to the hospital. Rain had fallen heavily during the concert, and puddles shone under the light from the red and white Emergency sign.

It had rained the first day Aaron walked through the sliding glass doors, four years before, not knowing how often he would return. The doors opened as he stepped towards them again, and closed behind him. The hospital swallowed the young pianist who, in a just universe, would have been out celebrating.

He asked a nurse to pump morphine into him. Seven hours later, another nurse found him asleep in his best suit, his shoes neatly laid beside the bed.

PART FOUR

'But there are worse things that can happen to an artist than to die young.'

Franz Schubert

30

LAST MAN STANDING

A year later, at 10.45 am on 28 September 2006, Charlie swept into the Prince of Wales operating theatre in his white monogrammed coat and dark blue scrub pants. Pulled low on his brow was a black surgical cap with the legend *Iowa Neurosurgery*, a gift from a visiting fellow. Only he knew that he was also wearing a new gift from his mother: red underpants with a yellow smiley face like a bullseye and the caption, *Mr Happy*. They were a replacement for his lucky socks, which had finally disintegrated. He wore sober black socks now. Five years after entering Aaron's brain, he was about to go in again.

'If I don't do the surgery, he's going to die within weeks,' he said. 'I can give him some time. He just wants to finish his composition. If it's going to take a year, I don't think I can promise him that, but if he can finish it in six weeks . . . That's if I don't kill him in surgery.'

Aaron had gradually lost the use of his legs that year as the tumours took over his spine, and at last conceded that his concert days were over. But, as his body failed, he simply adjusted his ambitions. Even now, he was uplifting company. Clear-eyed, amusing and curious about his friends' lives, he didn't complain about his failing health but always had headline news about his latest plans.

They formed and faded, and by mid-year had distilled into one grand idea. He intended to compose 'the Schubert piano concerto that Schubert never wrote'. Using musical computer software, he wanted to construct a piano concerto in the style of the great composer, who died at thirty-one without having written one of his own. As usual, Aaron did not make it easy for himself. He ordered bundles of Schubert recordings and sheet music. With Gail and Brian taking it in turns to care for him at Bondi, visits from palliative doctors and nurses, and friends bringing home-cooked meals, he sat at his computer, meticulously transcribing works such as the *Trout Quintet* and analysing the composer's musical patterns so that he could build on them. He even booked his friend Alexander Gavrylyuk, the Ukrainian pianist, to perform the finished piece in late 2007.

'Is this more difficult than just writing from your own head?' I asked.

'No . . . because there's nothing in my head,' he said.

Father Carola sent a string of rosary beads that Pope John Paul II had given him, and urged Aaron to be confirmed into the Catholic Church and make his first Holy Communion. Aaron agreed, mainly to please his friend, and Father Michael de Stoop, from St Mary's Cathedral in Sydney, performed the rites at his bedside. Aaron took Benedict as his confirmation name, after the new Pope, though he wished later he had chosen Michael, for the dragon-slaying saint. He could now receive another sacrament, the anointing of the sick. If the sacrament had any power, he was about to call on it.

'I hope I'm not going to die, but if it's meant to be . . .' That was as far as he went on the subject. Only with his grandparents, whose deaths he had long dreaded, could he talk about their shared destination and wonder who would get there first. With most friends, he wisecracked, 'I think I'll have to get used to a different sort of life – no jogging on the beach.' Gail prayed and Brian meditated at Aaron's side. Brian's years of absence in Thailand had given him a way to cope with this challenge. 'It's amazing how everything in our lives is preparing us for the present,' he said.

Experimental chemotherapy restrained the cancer for a few months but its toxicity soon outweighed its benefit. Bob Smee declared that Aaron's body could take no more radiation. Morphine and meditation eased his pain, but there were dead-ends in every direction. That was when Charlie Teo stepped up again.

Colleagues questioned why Charlie was going to operate in such a hopeless case. Even his latest registrar thought he was wrong. 'They have every right to say so,' he said. He had ignored such opposition before, of course, but this time he was weighed down by his own reservations. Aaron's surgery would be at the extreme end of his 'impossible' cases. What had been a large but clearly formed virgin tumour five years earlier had metastasised into pellets embedded throughout the brain tissue. Charlie would concentrate on the deepest and most dangerous growth. Whatever doubts he'd had last time, he had known surgery was the difference between certain death and possible cure. This time the gain was more difficult to see.

Charlie talked bluntly with Aaron. A lot of people thought it would be preferable to let the cancer take over and give a 'good, clean death', he said. Even he could see the sense in that. Aaron's answer was equally blunt: no way. Charlie was his last ally in keeping hope alive. He brushed aside the risks and began anticipating surgery as the way back to mental clarity. He didn't want sympathy. When Charlie commiserated that he must miss simple pleasures such as walking on the beach, he said, 'I've done that. All that matters is being able to compose music.' As the day approached, he wrote to Father Carola, 'There is a ten to fifteen per cent chance of death. So I put my faith in the Lord and ask for his guidance and protection.'

Charlie was in a bleak mood when he entered the theatre on the morning of surgery. Three of his patients had died in the previous twenty-four hours, one of them a two-year-old girl. He had been travelling and had hardly seen his family. Forcing himself into the cold spring day, he had cycled to Coogee beach, run six laps of the long curve of sand, pumped a hundred push-ups and a hundred sit-ups, and finished with a swim.

And now he had Aaron back on the table. Every other patient he'd first treated for a malignant tumour in 2001 had died over the ensuing years. As Aaron had put it, with black humour, he was the last man standing.

The surgical team had gently arranged the limp patient with a clamp holding his head upright. It would have been easier to operate if Aaron were face down but his spine couldn't take the stress. He was disguised under layers of gauze and adhesive bandage to protect his eyes, a sheet of plastic over his face and torso, and green sterile cloths over everything. Only his left big toe and the top of his head protruded. Charlie went to the light box and examined a set of brain scans taken the night before. The largest tumours stood out like light bulbs against the grey brain matter.

'Holy shit. Holy shit. They've got bigger . . . Look at that,' he said. He moved to the computer over the operating table, which would enable him to correlate the scans on its screen with points on Aaron's scalp and brain. 'This is futile,' he muttered. 'The disease has galloped away . . . This would have been a peaceful way for him to go.'

He cleared a patch of hair with his disposable razor, cut and parted the scalp and whirred into the skull with his burr-hole maker. 'We might go from hell to high water today,' he warned his crew. 'As soon as we open up, the whole brain's going to squeeze out. It's going to be very, very bad.' Lifting out a chunk of bone, he exposed the blood-smeared dura mater. Underneath, Aaron's brain throbbed with life.

Danger usually sharpened Charlie's senses but he was having trouble firing up. He opened a second hole in Aaron's skull to give double access to the buried tumour. Rather than the well-defined lump he had found the first time, this was like a conglomerate of five or six gumballs. When he pulled one away from the main mass, it set off a flood of bleeding. Soon he had three suckers trying to bail out the mess. Even though he had forecast a fifty per cent risk of death from blood loss as he began work that morning, he was shocked by the realisation that he could lose Aaron right then.

'Come on, Charlie,' he mouthed to himself. The reprimand worked. He focused, pushed on and finished the operation in less than four hours. Aaron had lost two and a half times his total blood volume, requiring transfusions of twelve litres. To get at the cancer, Charlie had removed an area of brain and destroyed any vestige of movement and sensation in Aaron's left leg. Most of the cancer remained. But the patient was alive.

'It was one of the worst days of my life,' Charlie said later.

'I almost lost him several times on the table. It was bloody, bloody, bloody.'

The medical system had always provided Aaron with ambulances, beds, first-rate doctors, surgery, radiation, chemotherapy, medicines and genuine care, at enormous cost to the state but none to him. It was impressive in the face of reports about strained staff and infrastructure. But as Aaron and Charlie fought their valiant losing battle, I had the uncomfortable suspicion that a quick death five years before might have been preferable for Aaron to this life of debilitating treatments.

'Aaron's tumour seems like one of the nastiest you could get because he had that respite and it has come back so furiously,' I said to Charlie one day.

'It's so funny hearing you say that,' he replied, 'because, to me, it's one of the better ones you can get. He's lived five years. Aaron has crammed so much into the last five years. He's had this great opportunity to live before he died, whereas other people don't have that. They die so quickly or they're so handicapped by their brain tumour that, even if they know they've only got one year to live, they can't live it because they can't talk or they can't see or they can't drive or they can't deliver their wisdom to their children, because their cognitive functions are flawed.

'Aaron's had the benefit of being functional and independent and clear-headed for five years. It's a great privilege to have had that. When I see the next young man with hemangiopericytoma, I'm going to treat him just as aggressively because I have seen that Aaron has enjoyed five great years. I'm not going to think, "Shit, this poor bastard's going to die anyway. I might as well let him die now."'

Gail Puckett had passed the day of her son's surgery more simply than she had five years earlier. No solitary prayers, no reaching out for the Holy Virgin, no clutching at babies. She had sat with Amy and a friend for hours of quiet meditation in a hospital garden near the operating theatre. Nervous but calm, she was numbed by a sense of resignation. Aaron was still acting courageously and the process he had gone through before his first operation of defining his purpose and deciding to live was threaded through his daily survival now and didn't need any special deliberations. Whatever he and his God said to one another, he kept private.

Recovery had become a relative term. Reluctantly, Aaron conceded that he needed more care than Gail and Brian and a relay of friends could give, and took up residence at the Sacred Heart Hospice at St Vincent's Hospital. Outside, crowds headed to the restaurants and bars of Oxford Street; boys leaned against the sandstone wall of the National Art School looking for business; addicts made their way to the methadone clinic and injecting room nearby. Life went on in all its vibrant, seedy rhythms. Inside the hospice, angular forms lay motionless, open-mouthed and white-haired under their sheets; a few sat in wheelchairs; staff broke up the shapeless days with deliveries of drugs and meals and efficient kindness; relatives and friends helped or hung around, swapping supportive smiles in the corridors. The atmosphere was quieter and, surprisingly, brighter than in many hospital wards, with extravagant vases of fresh flowers, windows onto the garden and no rules – a pleasant place to visit until you remembered that most of the patients would not be leaving.

It was no great surprise for Aaron's visitors to reach the room at the end of the corridor and find a young man in a wheelchair working on a computer, the stillness broken by a small field of energy. The cut on the back of his head was almost invisible and Aaron was impatient with questions about the surgery. He wanted to talk about music and the future. He didn't admit that he had left it too late to fulfil his dream of composing. But as he convalesced, he listened to the music he had recorded for his unfinished *Arc of Light* CD. If he could not compose, he would at least complete this task and honour the Australian musicians who had supported him.

Charlie was disappointed Aaron had moved into the hospice. He saw the decision to go there as a decision to die. With a brace and a wheelchair, visiting nurses and pain relief, he thought Aaron could live more independently, and perhaps longer, at home. Charlie's confidence was astonishing but he might as well have told Aaron to run a marathon. He was exhausted and in pain: stabbing attacks on the nerves in his feet; crippling morning head-aches; generalised pain that was only dulled by swamping his system with daily morphine doses as high as 1700 milligrams, then 1900 milligrams and 2200 and beyond. Ten milligrams could kill a healthy person. He was weakened by nausea and drowsi-ness and a gradual muddling of his thoughts. The palliative-care doctors tried to find a balance between comfort and consciousness.

One day, Gail stood in the corridor and watched a stream of young people flowing into the room next to Aaron's, where a man in his thirties was dying of cancer. 'I just wonder if I'll have to face this one day,' Gail said, her tears brimming but not spilling.

By mid-April 2007, fifteen bodies would be carried out of the room next door. Yet Charlie's intervention had pulled Aaron back from the brink and, within the confines of the hospice and his body, he lived as purposefully as ever. For his thirtieth birthday, on 11 February 2007, Gail organised a party in the garden. Although she was with him day and night, she was relieved of the hardest daily care by the nurses, who were fond of their longest staying resident. His room was home, office and salon, where music and friendship sustained him as always. As he told me one difficult day, 'This morning I called on the strength of all my friends to pull me back. I imagined them all here. That's one of my tricks.'

He found some comfort in the company of two fundamentalist Christians who drove up from Adelaide to promise healing through Christ. They had seen him on television in the *Australian Story* sequel soon after his second operation. In his usual open-minded way, Aaron read the Bible they gave him and talked about his friendship with Jesus. He would have accepted anyone's gift of salvation. But his real mission was on earth. With his computer by the bed, he worked like a man with a deadline.

The great pianist and conductor Daniel Barenboim has spoken about the tragedy of musical expression: notes emerge from silence, resonate as long as the musician strikes the key or the string, and then die. Music is as ephemeral as life itself. It is only by recording, he says, that musicians can 'preserve the unpreservable'.

After a brain scan that showed the rampaging growth of his cancer, Aaron decided to expand his project to producing a set of nine CDs that held every recording he had made in his short career. All his scattered performances – his compositions and improvisations, two Opera House concerts, the classics and the contemporary Australian music – would be organised into a musical biography. Even if he could never play again, his fans could hear him forever. Like a wounded general, he mounted a campaign to produce and sell *The Aaron McMillan Piano Collection 1995–2006*, and once again harnessed the collective energy of his friends. People stepped in to write notes, design packaging and publicise the finished work. His mother was a tireless assistant. Alan Jones, the Sydney broadcaster who had admired and promoted Aaron since his comeback from surgery in 2001, made the project possible by offering thirty-five thousand dollars to cover costs. He sat at Aaron's bedside, calling him 'Muhammad Ali' and urging him on: 'We're in the ring. We've got a fight on. Don't step out of the ring until the other bloke's knocked out. We'll make it to the fifteenth round.'

The collection was launched by Jones and Marie Bashir at the Sydney Conservatorium of Music on 19 April 2007. The evening was both a celebration and a sidelong glance at an approaching absence. 'What a fighter!' said Jones. 'One thing Aaron would want us to take from tonight – apart from a love of music, which he takes for granted – is the belief that he is going places and he's not leaving us.'

Aaron had videotaped his speech from bed and smiled down on the standing-room-only crowd from a vast screen. Wearing glasses and a red T-shirt, he was still a poised young man who joked about the daring music he had chosen to record at eighteen over his music teacher's suggestions of quieter, more modest pieces. But he seemed to be speaking from another dimension.

When I had asked him the day before the launch what he planned to do now the recordings were finished, he said, 'I can go on to my life's love of composing. That's what I absolutely promised myself. This finishes and that starts, the same day, and let's see how many weeks or months it takes me.'

31

NEVER SAY DIE

'I know I won't be able to do this for much longer, not these terrible, difficult cases,' Charlie told me as I drove him to Sydney airport in March 2007. He was flying to Florida to lecture on keyhole surgery and it was our only chance to talk. Working overseas for four months of the year, he seemed to be removing himself from the pressures of Australia and going where he was wanted. Once he left the country, he was unreachable.

'I've actually got a little bit depressed lately,' he said. He had seen Aaron in a wheelchair at his thirtieth birthday gathering a month earlier. But it wasn't Aaron who most upset him. Three patients had died in a week. One was a university student, a clever, sociable girl who kayaked and seemed to Charlie like a dream daughter. She had died just after her twenty-first birthday, almost two years after a diagnosis of a glioblastoma which she had followed with surgery, chemotherapy and experimental treatments. She had sent Charlie a Christmas card that said, in careful handwriting, 'You are an amazing person with a real gift. Not only did you perform surgery to put me on the road to recovery, but you came and told me after the surgery that it was me who had to beat this . . .'

Another was a seven-year-old boy whose brain stem tumour was of the truly inoperable, diffuse kind. After eight months of other failed treatments, his parents asked if Charlie could keep him alive a little longer. He agreed to remove some of the tumour. But the boy did not recover from surgery and Charlie had to advise his parents to turn off the ventilator and end his life. He felt guilty; his surgery had hastened rather than delayed death. Tears strangled his words as he explained the plan: they should not frighten the boy by saying goodbye but sit with him as he watched television and became sleepy with the morphine that would mask his pain.

Charlie emerged from his slump after a few weeks and some successful cases. He hadn't been depressed in a clinical sense, he rationalised, just had the edge taken off his spirit. It had given him a jolt, though, because 'depression and Charlie Teo just don't go together'. He thought depression was a bit wimpy. But he could feel the first signs of burn-out. His old mentor Ian Johnston had retired to a windswept beach in Tasmania, where he translated Chinese poetry. When Charlie invited him to come up to Sydney and watch him operate, Johnston declined. 'I'm enjoying being away from sickness,' he said. Charlie understood what he meant. He would turn fifty on 24 December, and Genevieve sensed that middle age was nibbling at his ego and his stamina. He responded by pushing himself harder and telling friends to anticipate 'the biggest party ever'.

Among his past patients was Barry Kelly, an airline pilot until he developed a brain tumour that doctors in Australia and Britain said was inoperable. He went to Charlie after his wife saw him on television, and had successful, though not curative, surgery. 'Because Charlie had faith in me, he extended my life,' he told me. 'You feel you can see his heart when he's talking.' Kelly gave a generous start-up donation to the Cure for Life Foundation. Four years later, he was turning forty-eight and asked Charlie to join him to walk the Kokoda Track, the 96-kilometre wartime path through Papua New Guinea's rugged terrain. It was just the challenge that Charlie needed.

During a medical examination required for the walk, a blood test showed Charlie to be pre-diabetic. He heard the diagnosis without shock. In medical school, he had learned that type 2 diabetes was hereditary and often skipped a generation. A grandparent on each side of his family had been diabetic. 'If you've got bad genes, there's nothing you can do about it,' he said. He did what he could. Instead of dipping into his lolly jar, he snacked on almonds and he intensified his exercise routine in preparation for the Kokoda trek. Within a few months, he had stripped seven kilograms from his frame and was declaring himself fitter than ever.

Charlie relaxed with as much energy as he worked. Genevieve had insisted on buying a beach house on the Central Coast, where they escaped for occasional weekends. Up there, he was like a ten-year-old kid, bushwalking, kayaking, swimming and playing on the sand with his daughters, who were sometimes exhausted by his enthusiasm.

'You can't help feeling invigorated when you're with him,' said the former Australian cricket captain Steve Waugh, who owned a neighbouring house. The two men shared another bond. Since retiring, Waugh had helped out with the Cure for Life Foundation, partly because he was attracted to Charlie's character.

When Jane McGrath, the wife of his fellow cricket star Glenn McGrath, was told in early 2006 that her breast cancer had metastasised into an inoperable brain tumour, Waugh gave her Charlie's phone number. Within a week, the tumour had been removed and, more than a year later, she was still in remission.

Waugh had no warning that his own wife, Lynette, would also need Charlie's help. She was taken ill suddenly with a cerebral haemorrhage in August 2006 and, as she was being rushed to the nearest hospital, Waugh called Charlie, who had the ambulance diverted to Prince of Wales. Charlie removed a blood clot that might have killed her. 'He's sensational, amazingly dedicated. He doesn't see what he does as a job,' Waugh told me as Lynette's health improved. He also liked Charlie's honesty. 'If there was bad news to be delivered, he gave it to us. He is optimistic without going over the top.'

Charlie's celebrity cases kept him in the news. When the famously abrasive radio personality Stan Zemanek was referred to him, neither man had heard of the other and each was struck by the other's brashness on the phone. But they also shared a 'fight tooth and nail' attitude. Zemanek came through a six-hour operation to remove the visible parts of his spreading glioblastoma multiforme and went back to work for six months, apparently a nicer man. He died in July 2007, fourteen months after being told that without surgery he had weeks to live.

Another well-known patient of Charlie's was Chris O'Brien, a fellow specialist in head and neck cancer who was familiar to the public through the television program *RPA*, which followed life at Royal Prince Alfred Hospital. In November 2006, he was diagnosed with a glioblastoma multiforme. A neurosurgeon at his own hospital, Michael Besser, operated, and gave him six to twelve months, even with radiotherapy and chemotherapy. Unwilling to accept his fate passively, in April 2007, O'Brien turned to Charlie. They had been acquaintances since working together as registrars and shared an attitude of aggressive optimism. With Besser's blessing, O'Brien submitted to several operations that year and, after a clear brain scan in June, was still living actively at the time of writing, in late 2007. It was long enough, at least, to learn that Frank Lowy, head of the Westfield shopping-centre empire, had donated ten million dollars towards O'Brien's dream, a comprehensive cancer research centre at the University of New South Wales.

Charlie's latest round of media attention brought a rare public response from the profession. In an interview with the television current affairs program *60 Minutes*, he was asked if he was 'the best' neurosurgeon for inoperable brain tumours. 'Well, I think I'm the best,' he said. He qualified that by saying every neurosurgeon had to believe the same thing in order to operate confidently, but he knew he'd made a diplomatic error and asked the producer to remove the line. Instead, it was used to promote the show. A newspaper advertisement in the form of an open letter from the president of the Neurosurgical Society of Australasia, Eric Guazzo, protested: 'The society is concerned that a recent media presentation may have caused the incorrect perception that the standard of neurosurgery available in Australia and New Zealand is not of the highest standard.' As for Charlie's reputation as a leader in endoscopic neurosurgery, Guazzo wrote: 'The suggestion during the interview that there is a reluctance to use or that this type of surgery is not widely available in Australia and New Zealand is erroneous and disparages the professional skill and knowledge available.'

Criticism was always offset by accolades, whether Charlie was receiving a Rotary Club award for vocational service or lecturing on keyhole surgery as a visiting professor at distinguished American universities such as Johns Hopkins, Stanford and the University of California, Los Angeles. As part of a specialist group that was preparing a book of national guidelines on cancer treatment, he was contributing to the chapter on brain tumours. Asked to chair the first annual general meeting of a New South Wales neuro-oncology group in December 2006, he invited as a speaker the like-minded American neurosurgeon Mitch Berger, who had been a pioneer of aggressive tumour surgery for twenty years. Charlie's results were showing that his patients with malignant glioma had a mean survival time of eighteen months after diagnosis, compared with eleven months worldwide. He hoped that if his Australian colleagues wouldn't listen to him, they might believe Berger.

The meeting went smoothly until Berger presented his argument. He said a major American study using data from many sources showed that complete removal of a low-grade tumour could give a patient an extra five to ten years of life. For high-grade tumours there was a shorter but still clear reprieve. The counter-arguments were that a tumour could turn malignant from only a few remaining cells and that surgery carried a risk of injury and could even stimulate malignancy.

A Sydney neurosurgeon in the audience challenged Berger with the hypothesis of a young mother suffering from a low-grade tumour. Surely, he said, Berger wouldn't operate if he might damage her and take her from her children when there was no guarantee of cure.

'No,' Berger conceded. 'You're right. That is a very difficult situation and I probably would not operate.'

But Charlie wouldn't let go so easily. 'Hang on, Mitch, you just told us a minute ago that you can prolong life and you can delay malignant transformation by taking out as much tumour bulk as you can. If this lady, for example, told you she'd be prepared to accept a deficit with radical surgery, knowing full well that it comes with no guarantee but it may prolong her life, you wouldn't offer it to her?'

Berger was trying to be diplomatic but he had to agree. 'Yes,' he said, 'I would offer it to her.'

The Sydney neurosurgeon stood and left the room.

Another doctor had voiced similar reservations to me almost four years earlier. 'Charlie's a bit of an entrepreneur,' he said. 'There's no doubt he's very well trained; his opinions are surgically aggressive but good. Overall, he's probably very good for neurosurgery. But you have to look at the reasons others have declined to operate. Some neurosurgeons thrive on the fact that they can achieve something that makes an MRI look better. If you realistically know a patient is going to die, you might ask, why offer surgery? It's a very difficult issue.'

Berger's view is that the majority of American neurosurgeons now accept aggressive surgery as beneficial and those who disagree are no longer in the mainstream. Australia is lagging. But he advised Charlie to have greater patience as he works to persuade his colleagues.

'My mission is not to proselytise,' Berger said. 'Our mission is to do cases and prove that the amount of tumour you remove does affect outcome, survival and quality of life. We've written articles about it but there are always people who don't want to believe it, because they can't do that kind of surgery. Charlie is going to keep on doing what he is doing and the proof is that people go to him from everywhere.'

In the seven years that Charlie had been a consultant to Sydney Children's Hospital, he had not received a single referral from

the other doctors there. Some of the people who had blocked his
job application when he arrived back from Arkansas were still
freezing him out. They would not directly state their opposition
but there was the usual stream of criticisms: Dr Teo did not
consult other doctors; Dr Teo didn't attend meetings; Dr Teo
behaved disrespectfully to the nurses; Dr Teo wore Hawaiian
shirts; Dr Teo was not a team player. When he gave a talk there
on advances in neurosurgery, one of the doctors' written reports
noted his 'unsurpassable arrogance'. Cath Hyam, who had run
Charlie's office all that time, heard from parents who had been
warned against seeing him because, according to other doctors,
he took excessive risks and left children as vegetables. She also
saw how most of his patients and their parents loved him and
were pleased with his results. In late 2006, worn down, Charlie
resigned from his position as a rostered visiting medical officer
at the hospital, retaining the right to operate there as an unpaid
honorary medical officer. His devotion to paediatric neurosurgery
had taken another beating. But he would not be beaten.

Most doctors refuse to criticise Charlie publicly, and most
parents are reluctant to tell their stories because they rely on the
Children's Hospital for follow-up treatment. However, a case
from farther afield illustrates the tensions.

Kate Hill was eight in 2005 when her turned-in eye led to a
diagnosis of a brain stem tumour. In the opinion of her neurosurgeon at the Women's and Children's Hospital in Adelaide,
Stephen Santoreneos, surgery was too dangerous; he prescribed
radiotherapy and chemotherapy, and gave her two years. But her
mother, Christine Warendorf, wanted to do more. Asking Santoreneos for other options, she was told of 'Dr Teo, an alternative
doctor in New South Wales', but was advised that her daughter
might return 'severely disabled, a child you would not want to

have around'. She was amazed to find on the internet that Charlie was a world-renowned neurosurgeon. She and Kate flew to Sydney. At his office, Charlie spoke directly and chatted about his children. Kate, along with her mother, was lifted out of depression. After warning that the risk was high and cure unlikely, Charlie operated. Kate emerged with slight weakness on one side requiring physiotherapy but returned to Adelaide happy and cheeky, able to go to school and play with friends. When she walked into Santoreneos' office and hugged him, he said it was a miracle to see her with so little deficit. Seven weeks later, however, she began to vomit and an MRI showed her tumour was growing quickly. Charlie recommended against further surgery. Over the next eight weeks, she lost the ability to swallow and finally fell unconscious. She died in hospital the following day, 8 January 2006, after being taken off her ventilator.

Was Charlie right or wrong to perform an operation that possibly shortened Kate's life? After he wrote about the case in an article for the International Society of Paediatric Neurosurgeons, Santoreneos placed his comment on the society's website. In part, the Adelaide surgeon said, 'I have been taught to choose my battles carefully and do not consider an anaplastic astrocytoma in this region a favourable lesion. The quality of life of this child was appalling and at a great financial cost an operation was performed which I think served no purpose other than to take the parents through a rollercoaster of emotions and the child to live her last days in hospital completely dependent.' He made some negative observations, which both Charlie and Warendorf said were untrue: that Charlie had recommended stopping chemotherapy, that Kate's quality of life was worsened by surgery, and that Charlie offered further surgery when her tumour recurred.

Warendorf happened upon Santoreneos' comments in early 2007, a year after they were published, and wrote a long, unsolicited response. The journal did not post her words and she did not hear from the society or the surgeon. But she eloquently expressed the experience of thousands of Charlie's patients.

'. . . Kate had seven amazing weeks in which we had a break emotionally from our situation. Kate was relieved, albeit for a time, and she felt personally cared for by Dr Teo. He always treated Kate as a special person worthy of his personal attention. She adored him and he made our experience more bearable. And I cannot emphasise how special and happy this time was for us. These are the memories that I treasure and make it easier for me and Kate's sisters to bear the burden of our grief . . . The only time we felt that Kate's quality of life was really "appalling" was when she was undergoing radio and chemotherapy . . . Dr Teo gave us a *break* from the horrific rollercoaster ride we were on. He looked after me as a mother living her worst nightmare . . . he was the only person who treated Kate as a person not a diagnosis. I felt confident with him, he was decisive, professional and honest. I felt I could make decisions with all the facts in front of me.

'I really feel that I can put my mind at rest [and] that I did everything possible to give my child a chance at life . . . Surely parents have a right to all the medical treatment options put before them from the outset so they can then make an informed decision and not be ushered into treatment they would like to avoid . . . I don't think it is for a doctor to "choose his battles carefully"; ultimately it was *my* battle and *my* decision to make about my child's treatment.

'Dr Teo gave Katie so much more than just brain surgery. He gave her the ability to laugh and smile again. He let her forget about her tumour – to not have to *be* her tumour. He gave me hope but at no stage was it false hope. I am eternally grateful to him for his attitude and expertise, his kindness and for lifting for a while the constant heaviness of our horrendous situation.

'Finally, doctors need to remember we are the parents of children who are fatally ill. This is a terrifying prospect. We require much care and consideration. We don't care about the egos of doctors but only about our children. We are hard work. We want all the answers and all the options, and every decision we make or is made for us affects the way we cope and grieve in the aftermath.'

32

REQUIEM

On Friday 11 May 2007, his room filled with family, friends and music industry officials, Aaron was presented with a Mo Award for his outstanding contribution to Australian music. Charlie attended, and Alan Jones handed over a crystal obelisk engraved with the figure of the vaudeville star Roy 'Mo' Rene. The trophy was too heavy for Aaron to hold but it made a perfect farewell gift. That day, his smile returned.

Visitors came over the weekend and, though talking was difficult, he asked each one, 'How are you?' Some could sense his fear of dying; some saw acceptance. But it was not the subject he wanted to discuss. He spoke to his publicist, Philippa Drynan, about their campaign to sell his CDs and sent her away with the words 'We have a lot to do.' His final conversations on Sunday were about music, with the pianist Gerard Willems, who had known him since he was eighteen, and the director of the Sydney Conservatorium, Kim Walker. Willems read aloud the Mo citation three times at Aaron's request and Walker assured him that he could go when he was ready, taking pride in his achievements. He must have agreed.

On Monday 14 May, a nurse woke Gail at 3 am. 'Aaron is taking his last breaths,' he said. She ran down the hall of the hospice from the family room where she had been sleeping but, by the time she reached Aaron's side, he had died. His body already had the translucence of marble. The creases had cleared from his face and his long fingers stretched out lightly on the sheet.

A heavy fog shrouded the city as Gail spread the news by phone and switched on the CD player to fill the room with Aaron's music as his last visitors arrived. She wondered how, in all the time she had spent with her son, she had not been there to ease his parting moments. At ten o'clock the previous night, she had kissed his cheek and said, 'Goodnight, sweet prince,' as she always did, not suspecting she was saying goodbye. She believed he had waited until Sunday, Mother's Day, was over. Or perhaps it is simply easiest for the dying to slip away in the solitude of night.

Aaron's determination had created an illusion that life in the hospice could go on indefinitely. But he had been letting go since the launch of his music collection. It was just as Charlie had said: he had held on until his task was done and he hadn't the strength to start another.

The young pianist's death made the Monday morning news bulletins and quickly spread around the world. An intimate prayer vigil was held on Thursday evening in the vaulted crypt of St Mary's Cathedral. Aaron's body lay in an open coffin, his cheeks and lips pinkened, a prayer book in his hand and the *Live strong* yellow band around his wrist. People told stories about the man, or the boy, they loved. Sylvie Renaud-Calmel's soprano and the deep notes of a cello played by his childhood friend Johanna Fluhrer resounded off the mosaic floors, filling every listener's hollow centre.

The week of public mourning ended on Friday with a grand funeral at St Mary's. The date, as Father Joseph Carola pointed out, was 18 May, the birthday of Pope John Paul II. A wild rainstorm interrupted the city's drought that morning and dripping figures crowded into the cathedral pews as if for a state funeral or a concert. Some important people were missing: Charlie was operating in Tokyo. Genevieve spoke for him, recalling how he had conceived the Cure for Life Foundation while paddling a kayak with Aaron, a considerate, beautiful, talented young man, who did not discuss girls and motorbikes but wanted to help the world. Father Carola had hoped to conduct the mass but his superiors had refused him permission to leave Rome, where he had academic duties and was about to take his final vows. Instead, he had sat up late into the night writing a sermon, which was delivered by Father Michael de Stoop. In it, Father Carola recalled how Aaron's spiritual awakening had begun with their friendship and continued until a few hours before his death, when they prayed the Hail Mary together over the phone.

'Aaron,' he wrote, 'while your "Schubert" piano concerto must go unfinished, your life in the Lord has become your masterpiece. In cooperating with the abundant grace which God bestowed upon you, you have composed in your very being a glorious hymn of praise unto the Lord.'

As she had so often, the Governor found a place in her schedule for Aaron, this time to deliver a eulogy that celebrated 'a young Australian with extraordinary zest for life and dignity, who touched our lives in countless ways'. She ended by reading a few lines that Gail had written about her son. He had, she said, grown in wisdom and patience over the past three years as one would expect of someone who had lived a much longer life. Marie Bashir's voice faltered at Gail's last line: 'Aaron will be deeply missed but through the legacy of his beautiful music he will stay in our hearts forever . . . Goodnight, sweet prince.'

The St Mary's Cathedral Choir sang and Alan Jones wept as the twelve-year-old violinist Alison Laurens played Jules Massenet's beautiful 'Meditation' from *Thaïs*. Six solemn young men – Aaron's brother, Andrew, his cousins John and Carlos Robinson, his schoolmates Sebastian Adams and Troy Henderson, and the cricketer Elliot Bullock – carried the coffin past the *Pietà*, a copy of the Michelangelo sculpture with Mary's upturned marble hand forever questioning her loss. A small group gathered at the Catholic section of Macquarie Park Cemetery as Aaron's body was interred. The rain stopped but a layer of bruised cloud looked as if it might pelt the scene with hail. 'Hail Mary!' said Roselle, puncturing the solemnity of the place. A simple gravestone, laid later between two white camellia trees, repeats Schubert's epitaph, 'Here music has buried a treasure . . .'

It was a day of sorrow, relief and unexpected joy. Aaron's wake was held at the Woollahra home of Michelle Purves, a friend of Peter Crisp. Gail's eyes shone as she led a conga line through the elegant Victorian rooms, waving sparklers and singing 'Happy Birthday' to her husband. Giles had given his wife gentle support in exchange for neglect while Aaron needed her more than he did. Now he and everyone else, awash with emotion, deserved a moment's celebration. The clouds evaporated and late-afternoon sun lit the party. Gail and Brian sat down together with a cup of tea as evening fell along with a strange kind of peace. Aaron would have smiled.

Epilogue

I knew the book I was writing had changed when I came home with my Saturday shopping on 10 January 2004 to two telephone messages. I had been anticipating the news for longer than I wanted to admit. In a dream two nights earlier, I was lying on a hospital trolley and being rushed down a corridor to an operating theatre. The overhead lights flashed by, the doors closed and I could feel the weight of the anaesthetic. I woke just before oblivion crushed me.

The messages from Aaron and Charlie asked me to ring them urgently. Aaron told me about the previous day's scans, which had revealed the recurrence of his cancer, this time in his neck, after two years' apparent remission. Speaking from his grand-parents' retirement home on the Central Coast, where he had gone looking for some mental stillness, he said, 'At least I'm lucky it's nothing like the last one. It's not a tumour the size of a cricket ball wrapped around the vein of Galen. It's in the tissue of my neck and there's absolutely no risk of death from surgery.' He ended a little less brightly: 'Say a prayer for me.'

Charlie was finishing an emergency surgery when he answered his mobile phone. His voice echoed in the tiled theatre and he let out a long moan. 'Susan, have you heard?' He had yet to read the sparse literature on metastasising hemangiopericytoma but he quietly feared for Aaron. 'This one's too close to home,' he said as he went back to stitching his patient's head.

At first it seemed I couldn't continue with the book. My heroes had taken a fall and their happy ending had unravelled. It felt heartless even to think of Aaron and Charlie as subjects; they were friends in need of emotional support. But as time went by I saw that Aaron was facing this challenge with the same determined optimism that had carried him through the first shock of his illness and had driven his musical career. When I visited him in hospital soon after the new diagnosis, he joked to a friend, 'Susan said the book was too short so I thought I'd give her another chapter.' His story was still an inspiration and our work gave him a purpose.

Like many others around him, for a long time I was willing to believe he could still beat the disease through some miracle of medicine, providence or sheer desire. Charlie, too, was a continuing source of stories, uplifting or sombre but always engrossing. While Aaron was more than a patient – he had become a friend, an ambassador, an advertisement – Charlie had to extend his concern to new patients every day. I realised that Aaron's experience was now a more realistic case study of the neurosurgeon's work. Yet, it also illustrated Charlie's philosophy: he would fight on with conviction as long as surgery could bring any benefit.

*

Part-friend, part-observer, I was among dozens of people who visited Aaron in the final months. On the day he died, his mother rang me at four o'clock in the morning and by 4.30 I was sitting with her at her son's side, holding his hand and drinking tea from one of the hospice's best cups. Aaron had vacated his gaunt, beautiful young body but he was still a forceful presence in the room. Hearing his music brought tears, as it still does, but mainly I felt exhausted relief that his struggle had ended and disbelief that he was gone.

Much of my grieving was done earlier, as I gradually accepted his decline. When I followed him into the operating theatre where Charlie probed his brain for the second time it was like stepping into a scene from my book. Aaron didn't see me cry but I howled after I left the hospital that day. I cried for his suffering, his bravery and his unfulfilled hopes, and for the inexorable march of death into all our lives.

Other people came to the hospice after he died, some of them trembling with sobs, and Gail was their comforter. Her tears would come later, once she had dealt with the formalities of death and retreated to her home in Brisbane. Though no one would wish a mother this tragedy, she'd grown visibly in strength and tenderness over the year or more when she cared almost full-time for Aaron. In that time she had also found the clarity of mind to finish her degree in education and help her daughter through her final school exams. But her main concern was to enjoy the bond with her son. Aaron's illness, she told me, had taken them on a spiritual journey together and death would not separate them.

She gave Aaron a Catholic funeral, she said, 'because he needed to make up his mind to be in one camp and prepare for the next world. It was too late to take on Buddhism. He was baptised

Catholic and his Catholic grandparents prayed for him every day. Then we met Father Carola: how many signs do you need?'

Four months after the funeral, when Gail visited the cemetery in Sydney to lay a cluster of springtime jasmine on Aaron's freshly engraved plaque, she felt a stab of injustice that all the other new graves were for people in their eighties. She planned to create a memorial garden at home where could sit quietly to meditate and build a different relationship with him; a consecrated site was a powerful place for memories and tears.

Her emotions rose and plummeted as she tended her garden, went back to part-time teaching, and spent time with her husband, children and parents. She was also occupied with settling Aaron's affairs: she lived among piles of letters, photographs and bills. He had cleared some old debts in his last weeks and Gail paid some more. 'I feel I'm helping myself in healing his past and helping him sort this out,' she said. Many of us knew that his ambitions, unmatched by financial sense, had caused him to spend irresponsibly – always looking dreamily towards the end of the next rainbow – and his sickness had left him unable to make amends. One of his most loving friends worried that if he had lived he might have ended up destitute, while another pointed out that Wagner always owed money too. Perhaps Aaron really was meant to have a fleeting, Peter Pan life. As his kinder-garten teacher told Gail a few months after his death, even as a small child it was clear that he stepped lightly on the earth.

Among the many tributes to Aaron's life is a string quartet by George Palmer, a judge of the New South Wales Supreme Court as well as a composer. While visiting Aaron in the hospice, Palmer was impressed by his calm creative energy in the face of mortality. 'This is what we will remember Aaron for and this is what he would have thought of his own life,' he told me. 'This sort of artistic energy survives death, you know. Where a positive life is led, that positive energy continues in others, so the music ends on a very affirmative note.' His title, *Not Going Quietly*, was about all of us. 'We should never go quietly in a sense of defeat. You can go with peace, you can go with acceptance, but that's not a sense of defeat.'

The last time I spoke to Charlie Teo before finishing this book was by telephone in September 2007. He was at Sydney Airport, about to leave the country for three weeks, and was on crutches after being knocked off his motorbike by a P-plate driver. The pain from three broken bones in his foot was excruciating. But there was no slowing down.

At London's Heathrow Airport he was scheduled to see eight patients for consultations before heading to the annual meeting of the International Society for Paediatric Neurosurgery in Liverpool, followed by a meeting of the American Association of Neurological Surgeons in San Diego and a booked-out course in Portland, Oregon. He was just back from Indonesia, where he had signed an agreement with a private hospital in Jakarta to start a pro bono program of surgery and teaching like those he had run for ten years in Peru and two years in Vietnam. With his fiftieth birthday imminent, he said pro bono work was his priority for the next phase of his career.

'It's got to the point where it's hard to get an appointment with me in Sydney. But I'm doing thirty brain tumours a month, which is a lot... Hey,' he added, 'do you want to know the latest?'

In Brisbane a week earlier, he had delivered the fiftieth E.S. Meyers Memorial Lecture, a public event organised by the

University of Queensland Medical Society in honour of a founding father of the medical faculty. Charlie was flattered to join a list of speakers that included the mountain climber Sir Edmund Hillary, heart-transplant surgeon Dr Victor Chang, cricketer Imran Khan and plastic surgeon Dr Fiona Wood. Alistair Hamilton, a second-year medical student and convenor of the 2007 lecture, had nominated Charlie after meeting a woman who was grateful for his surgery on her son's brain tumour which had extended his life by several months to his seventh birthday.

However, during the lead-up to the lecture, a fracas broke out behind the scenes. The Neurological Society of Australasia sent a letter protesting that Charlie Teo was an inappropriate speaker. This was the same organisation whose Queensland-based president, Eric Guazzo, took out a newspaper advertisement after Charlie appeared on *60 Minutes*. Some Brisbane neurosurgeons personally expressed their discontent to the head of the medical school, Professor David Wilkinson, but they were countered by more senior figures who argued against interference in the students' plans. There were no sound reasons given for the opposition and the student organising committee decided to go ahead.

On 31 August a thousand people packed the hall for the lecture, which Charlie called 'What doesn't kill you makes you stronger'. No critics spoke up in the fifty-minute question time. Afterwards Charlie stayed out late at a pub, talking to students and drinking water, and next day he gave a workshop on leadership in medicine.

'It was a massive success,' said Hamilton. 'The students thought he was awesome and Derek Meyers, the son of E.S. Meyers, told me that he was impressed with both the lecture and Charlie himself.'

No matter how established and successful Charlie becomes, and how often his techniques are vindicated, it seems he will always face hostility. After five years' watching him work, interviewing him and many other doctors, I understand why he infuriates some, but I have neither seen nor heard evidence of any actions that reduce my respect and affection for him. Like Aaron, he generates joyful energy, and his charisma radiates out through ever-growing circles of patients, students, neurosurgeons and other supporters.

Is he any less heroic for not saving Aaron's life? It was a huge blow, of course, to admit he didn't have all the answers. There were times I wondered if his focus on preserving Aaron's musical abilities stopped him from taking steps, such as immediate radiotherapy, that might have helped or even cured him. But he and others made it clear that this strange cancer was probably in Aaron's system before his diagnosis and was unlikely to be halted. I questioned whether Charlie had given Aaron the 'false hope' of which he was so often accused. But I look back to interviews I did with both of them from the beginning and see the unambiguous truth. At Charlie's home in March 2003, his daughter Nikki asked the question for me: 'Daddy, didn't Aaron have a "maligament" brain tumour?'

He replied, 'Aaron does have a malignant brain tumour. It's a hemangiopericytoma, a very rare type. He knows.'

Despite the small warning voice in the back of his head, Aaron shared Charlie's attitude that while he was alive he would live with gusto. Charlie's only mistake was in thinking that any regrowth of the tumour would be in Aaron's brain and could be removed again. He knows a lot more now.

In September 2007, I asked how he looked back on Aaron's illness and treatment and his answer was hardly different from a year earlier. 'I woke up the other day thinking about him,' he said. 'I feel good about what we did for Aaron and that he could achieve all the things he wanted. Without detracting from the impact Aaron had on me and the greatness of Aaron, he's just another patient who died. They all have a huge impact on me.'

Charlie is not a superhero or a saint. He once told me that if he had brain cancer he couldn't be sure he'd be as brave as his patients often are. But I believe he is heroic, like all neurosurgeons, for simply carrying on every day in good spirits with their life-and-death work. They are astronauts venturing to inner rather than outer space.

Every year about 1500 Australians are diagnosed with a malignant brain tumour. Some 1100 die; and the numbers are growing. Fundraising for the Cure for Life Foundation is expected to reach two million dollars in 2008 and recent grants support several genetic research projects.

Amid all the noble exploration and technical talk, an understanding of what causes brain tumours and a cure seem as far off – or perhaps just as close – as a comprehensive explanation of how a brain animates a conscious, creative individual. For all my observations, reading and discussions with neurosurgeons, neurologists and neuroscientists, I still can't believe that human beings are wholly contained in the bowl of porridge inside our heads. Pieces of the physical picture clarify, but some intangible, scientifically inexplicable element seems necessary to give us our spark. I'll accept the scientists' answers if they come and I will celebrate the day when medicine can save the Aaron McMillans of the future. But as thinking, dreaming, striving creatures, we will always need a touch of mystery and I'm content with that.

BIBLIOGRAPHY

Books

Carter, Rita, *Mapping the Mind*, Phoenix, London, 2000.

Chopra, Deepak, MD, *Quantum Healing: Exploring the Frontiers of Mind/Body Medicine*, Bantam Books, New York, 1990.

Epstein, Fred, MD and Horwitz, Joshua, *If I Get to Five: What Children Can Teach Us about Courage and Character*, Henry Holt, New York, 2003.

Goodman, Linda, *Linda Goodman's Sun Signs*, Pan Books, London, 1972.

Greenfield, Susan, *The Human Brain: A Guided Tour*, Phoenix, London, 1998.

Hazzard, Shirley, *The Great Fire*, Virago Press, London, 2003.

Kleihues, Paul and Cavenee, Webster K. (eds), *Pathology and Genetics of Tumours of the Nervous System: World Health Organization Classification of Tumours*, IARC Press, Lyon, 2000.

Nuland, Sherwin B., *How We Live: The Wisdom of the Body*, Vintage, London, 1998.

Pinker, Steven, *How the Mind Works*, W.W. Norton, New York, 1997.

Ramachandran, V.S. and Sandra Blakeslee, *Phantoms in the Brain*, Fourth Estate, London, 1998.

Ratey, Jon, *A User's Guide to the Brain*, Abacus, New York, 2002.

Rosen, Charles, *Piano Notes: The Hidden World of the Pianist*, Allen Lane-Penguin, London, 2003.

Sacks, Oliver, *Musicophilia: Tales of Music and the Brain*, Picador, London, 2007.

Sylvester, Edward J., *The Healing Blade: A Tale of Neurosurgery*, Beck Press, Tempe, Arizona, 1997.

Thorwald, Jurgen, *The Triumph of Surgery*, Thames and Hudson, London, 1960.

Vertosick, Frank T., Jr, MD, *When the Air Hits Your Brain: Tales of Neurosurgery*, W. W. Norton, New York, 1996.

Articles and reports

'Music to Their Brains', *The Australian*, 30 October 2004.

'Brain Surgeon Works 100 Hours a Week', *The Sun Herald*, 11 December 1988.

'U.S. Home to World's Best Neurosurgeon', University of Arkansas for Medical Sciences, 23 February 2000, at www.newswise.com/articles/2000/2/SURGERY.UAM.html

'M. Gazi Yasargil: Neurosurgery's Man of the Century' by John M. Tew Jr MD, *Neurosurgery*, 45 (5), November 1999.

'Gone But Not Forgotten: Renaissance of the Harvey Cushing Brain Tumor Registry' by Christopher J. Wahl, Yale School of Medicine, at www.neurosurgery.org/cybermuseum/tumor registryhall/wahl.html

SUNY Buffalo study on the physical and psychological effects of music on surgeons, Journal of the American Medical Association, September 1994.

'This Is Stan Zemanek' by Jane Cadzow, *Good Weekend*, 25 November 2006.

Television and radio

'Playing for Time', *Australian Story*, ABC-TV, 27 September 2001.

'The Trouble with Charlie', *Australian Story*, ABC-TV, 5 May 2003.

'His Hour Upon the Stage', *Australian Story*, ABC-TV, 9 October 2006.

Barenboim, Daniel, Reith Lectures 2006, Lecture 1, 'In the Beginning Was Sound', at www.bbc.co.uk/radio4/reith2006

ACKNOWLEDGEMENTS

My deepest thanks go to Aaron McMillan and Charlie Teo for allowing me to enter their lives and tell their stories. I only wish Aaron was able to read the finished book.

Many other people – too many to name – contributed generously to my understanding of my characters and of neurosurgery, music, religion and other subjects that run through the book.

I am especially grateful to Aaron's mother, Gail Puckett, and his father, Brian McMillan, and to other members of his family, who warmly accepted my presence during the most difficult period of their lives and helped me in many practical ways.

Thanks to Aaron's friends, professional contacts, doctors and other carers who told me their piece of his story. Sharing this experience made it bearable and often fun. Thank you to Simon Creedy for his photographs, Roselle Gowan for her painting and David Wansbrough for his poetry.

My thanks, too, to Charlie's wife, Genevieve Teo, and to their daughters, Alexandra, Nicola, Katie and Sophie, who were welcoming and gracious about my demands on his time. Many of Charlie's friends, colleagues and others in his medical network in Australia, the United States and elsewhere talked to me, which I greatly appreciate. I also thank his patients, some of whom are no longer alive, and their families, who agreed it was important to record their histories.

It has been a pleasure to work with Pan Macmillan and I thank the two Picador publishers – Nikki Christer for her early belief in my book and her patience; and her successor, Rod Morrison, for his enthusiasm and skill in helping shape the manuscript; also, Sarina Rowell for her sharp-eyed, sympathetic editing.

I could not have written the book without steady support from my husband, Paul Sheehan, in particular, and from my family, friends and workmates. Thanks to everyone who asked, 'How's the book going?' and listened to the answer.

Grateful acknowledgement is given for permission to reproduce extracts from the following works:

Linda Goodman's Sun Signs, Pan Macmillan, London, © Linda Goodman 1972

V.S. Ramachandran and Sandra Blakeslee, *Phantoms in the Brain*, reprinted by permission of HarperCollins Publishers Ltd © V.S. Ramachandran and Sandra Blakeslee 1998

Oliver Sacks, *Musicophilia: Tales of Music and the Brain*, Picador, London, 2007 © Oliver Sacks 2007

John M. Tew Jr MD, 'M. Gazi Yasargil: Neurosurgery's Man of the Century', *Neurosurgery*, 45 (5), November 1999, p. 1010